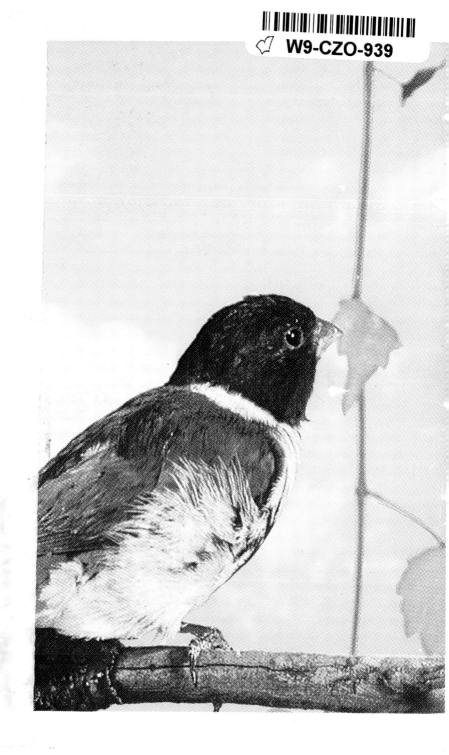

CONTENTS:

Front endpapers: Alario finches. Photo courtesy of Vogelpark Walsrode.
Back endpapers: Sierra parakeet. Photo courtesy of Vogelpark Walsrode.
Title page: Peach-faced lovebird. Photo by Dr. Herbert R. Axelrod.

Photo Credits:
Harry V. Lacey: 7; L. Arnall: 26, 27, 31, 48, 59, 80, 82, 83 (bottom); Dr. Herbert R. Axelrod: 6, 11, 14, 15, 23, 30, 70, 71, 74, 81; Miceli Studios: 8, 16 (top); William Allen: 16 (bottom); John Daniel: 10; Ralph Cooper: 18; Barbara Kotlar: 19; Glen S. Axelrod: 21, 49, 90; Gary Lilienthal: 22; Julie Sturman: 66, 86 (bottom); Ray Hanson: 67, 91; Tony Silva: 87; Vince Serbin: 58; Dr. Gerald R. Allen: 75; G.J.M. Timmerman: 60.

ISBN 0-87666-897-X

Distributed in the UNITED STATES by T.F.H. Publications, Inc., 211 West Sylvania Avenue, Neptune City, NJ 07753; in CANADA by H & L Pet Supplies Inc., 27 Kingston Crescent, Kitchener, Ontario N2B 2T6; Rolf C. Hagen Ltd., 3225 Sartelon Street, Montreal 382 Quebec; in ENGLAND by T.F.H. (Great Britain) Ltd., 11 Ormside Way, Holmethorpe Industrial Estate, Redhill, Surrey RH1 2PX; in AUSTRALIA AND THE SOUTH PACIFIC by Pet Imports Pty. Ltd., Box 149, Brookvale 2100 N.S.W., Australia; in NEW ZEALAND by Ross Haines & Son, Ltd., 18 Monmouth Street, Grey Lynn, Auckland 2 New Zealand; in SINGAPORE AND MALAYSIA by MPH Distributors Pte., 71-77 Stamford Road, Singapore 0617; in the PHILIPPINES by Bio-Research, 5 Lippay Street, San Lorenzo Village, Makati, Rizal; in SOUTH AFRICA by Multipet Pty. Ltd., 30 Turners Avenue, Durban 4001. Published by T.F.H. Publications Inc., Ltd., the British Crown Colony of Hong Kong. THIS IS THE 1983 EDITION.

BIRD DISEASES

HEINZ-SIGURD RAETHEL

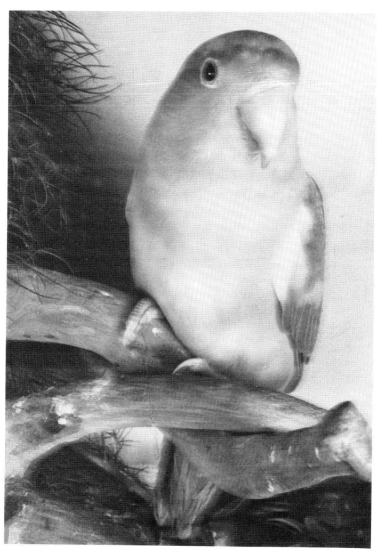

Translated by CHRISTA AHRENS

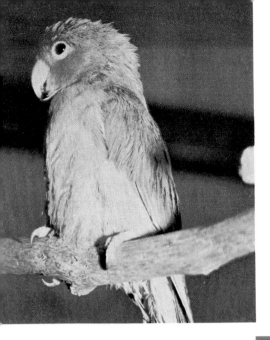

Left: The health of a bird that continues to look like this is questionable.
Below: The cut-throat finches shown (adults and juveniles) evidence the alertness, robustness and tight feathering of healthy birds.

*Look
Before
You
Buy*

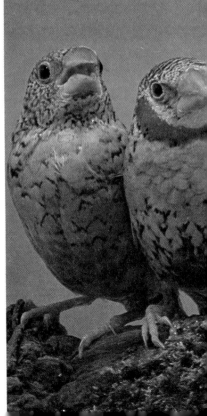

All too often a potential bird fancier buys a bird and then finds it dies on him. This may be so upsetting as to put him off keeping birds for the rest of his life. Fortunately one can safeguard against selecting a death candidate by looking out for a number of important points. After choosing a particular bird in the shop, one should not buy it right away but should step back and watch the animal's behavior from a distance. A healthy bird presents smooth, close-lying feathers and takes a lively interest in its surroundings. If the bird flutters about anxiously when one comes near it, then this is a good sign and in fact the rule where newly caught birds are concerned. If, on the other hand, there is a bird which sits about quietly with its feathers ruffled, then that apparent "tameness" gives little cause for pleasure. In virtually

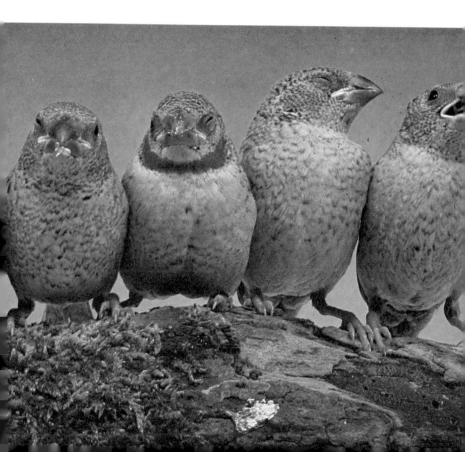

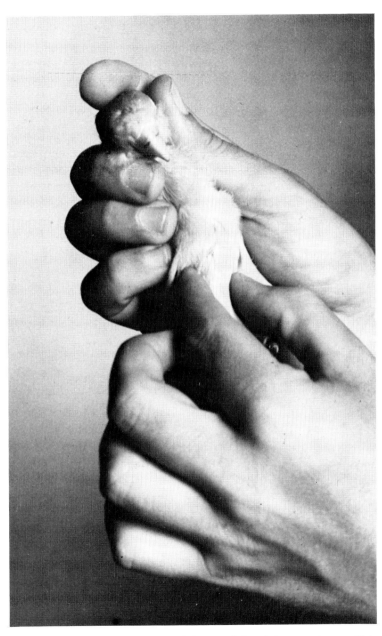

You should examine each bird you intend to purchase. This lovebird's breast is being felt to determine whether the bird is well nourished.

every case this will be a sick bird which has already become indifferent to its environment. Conversely, the wildly fluttering bird usually settles down and becomes less shy within just a few weeks from when it was purchased, as soon as it gets used to its new surroundings and has recognized its keeper as the provider of food.

Another point to make sure of before buying a bird is that the animal is properly nourished. A novice reluctant to touch the bird because he is not yet sure how to pick it up should ask the dealer to hold it and should then feel the pectoral musculature with his thumb and index finger. If the keel of the breastbone projects narrowly and sharply like a ship's keel, then the bird is emaciated and must on no account be purchased. In a healthy bird the musculature on both sides of the keel of the breastbone is so well developed that only a narrow hard partition can be felt between the two portions of muscle.

Further, it is important to examine the condition of the vent feathers. The feathers in this area must be as clean, dry, soft, and fluffy as elsewhere on the body. If they are stained and matted by liquid feces, the bird is suffering from some sort of intestinal inflammation.

On the other hand, the plumage of a bird one intends to purchase need not necessarily be complete. Damaged primary feathers, broken or missing tail feathers, or even a bald patch on the forehead is not a sign of disease but is very likely due to the bird's restless behavior in transit and inside the dealer's cage. Sometimes parts of the primaries are trimmed with scissors to prevent very anxious birds from throwing themselves about in a panic and doing themselves injury. Where parrots are concerned, however, individuals with missing feathers should be shunned as they may well be self-pluckers, an undesirable habit that is very difficult to cure.

Adhesions around the edges of the beak so often seen in fruit-eating species such as leaf birds, tanagers, sugar birds, and bulbuls are not pathological changes but merely bits of banana, fig, and orange that have remained attached after the birds have fed on large pieces of fruit. If the birds are given smaller pieces of fruit which are easier for them to handle, the feathers in the beak area will soon revert to normal.

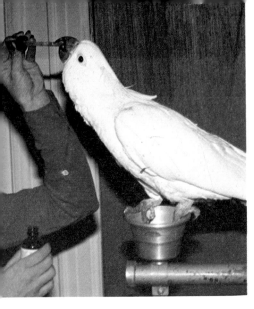

Left: Not all sick birds will take medicine or dietary supplements from an eyedropper as easily as this greater sulphur-crested cockatoo. Using a plastic, not glass, eyedropper is safer with strong-billed birds. **Below:** Ill birds should be isolated so they do not infect others in your collection. Many medicines can be administered in water via the tube drinker.

Care of the Sick Bird

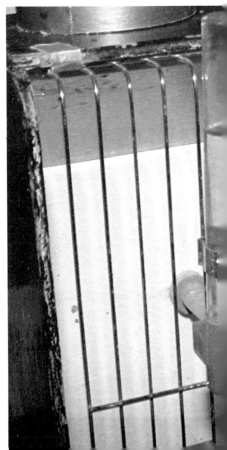

What action does the keeper take when he notices that one of his birds has become ill? A case of illness is certain to occur at some time or other, and the keeper should be prepared for it at all times. A small cage or, better still, a special "hospital cage" should always be in readiness. An infra-red heater should not be absent either, nor a small first-aid box for the birds containing at least a pair of forceps, scissors, some tincture of iodine, a coagulant powder, and an antibiotic. If these items are readily available at all times, the keeper will be able to cope with quite a few bird diseases himself.

In most cases the sick bird will ruffle its feathers and sit about like a sad ball of fluff. If the animal is alone in its cage and the

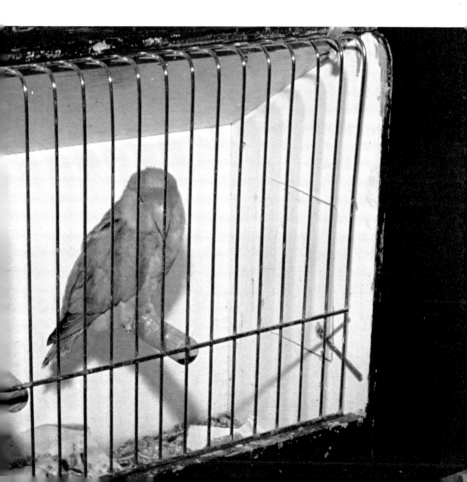

cage is not too big, it may be left inside. In all other cases, the patient is transferred to a small box cage with a wire mesh front or to an all-wire cage which (apart from the front, which must be left open) is covered with a cloth. In front of the cage we place an infra-red radiator of 250 watts. The heat produced by this radiator should keep the temperature inside the cage at 35-40°C.

Considerable advantages in the treatment of a sick bird are offered by a hospital cage. The typical hospital cage is 35 cm long, 17 cm deep, and 30 cm high. By means of a grate, it is divided into a larger upper and smaller lower compartment. The lower part – which is about 10 cm high – is lined over all the inside with asbestos. The back wall is fitted with three electric light bulbs, each of which is operated by an outside switch. The two narrow sides are each equipped with three strips of wood fixed horizontally above each other. The top one supports the frame for the grate, on the middle one rests a frame with taut canvas, and the bottom strip holds an asbestos plate with numerous holes 2 cm in diameter. The upper compartment of the cage, in which the patient lives, is fitted with a pane of glass that projects above and is easily removed. The walls contain a door, two openings for the porcelain seed and water cups, and – not far below the ceiling – several air-holes which can be opened and closed by means of a sliding panel. Two perches are screwed into the back wall, and a thermometer is fixed to one of the side walls.

Where the cage is heated with light bulbs of 40, 25, and 15 watts, trial and error will establish which produce the most favorable temperatures. When the cage is in use the heat moves through the holes in the asbestos plate, cloth, and grid into the upper compartment of the cage, where the temperature should remain constant at a maximum of 40°C. The cloth frame fitted below the grid serves to catch the droppings. The grid can readily be removed if the flap at the front is opened. When the bird is on the road to recovery, the temperature is reduced gradually to prevent the animal from catching a chill. The drink of a bird suffering or convalescing from an internal disease that has not been identified precisely should consist of an antibiotic such as Aureomycin dissolved in water.

Unfortunately, the behavior of a bird with an internal ailment seldom points to a specific diagnosis, and neither do particular signs of illness indicate any specific focus; they can, in fact, have many different causes. Difficulty in breathing and rhythmical opening of the beak, for instance, are most frequently caused by a circulatory weakness which may be due to bacterial and viral infections. More or less identical symptoms are also observed in worm infestations of the trachea, fungus diseases, pneumonia, colds, thyroid enlargement in the budgerigar, and egg-binding. Head-shaking with a discharge of mucus, for example, occurs in tracheal worm infestation, colds, and "soft crop" (crop infection).

Diarrhea may be the result of a chill, coccidiosis, B-hypovitaminosis, pseudotuberculosis, or a paratyphoid infection. Fits generally occur when there is a vitamin B deficiency, but they are also seen after cerebral concussion and in cases of vitamin E deficiency, ergot poisoning, and chronic insecticide poisoning.

A number of infectious diseases in birds result in the formation of crusty deposits on the skin and abnormal growths of the outer layer of the skin. In cnemidocoptic mange (or scaly face) scabs and crumblike growths of a peculiar brittle nature form particularly in the facial and cloacal region. The horny parts of the beak and the feet are also affected by these mites. Very similar are the crusty deposits seen in certain fungus infections of the skin known as favus. These, too, frequently appear in the facial region. As distinct from mange, however, they are not of a brittle consistency. Bird pox pustules occur most prominently on the skin around the edges of the beak and on the eyelids. They start off as pin-head sized little yellow pustules which later burst and develop into dark brown crusts. Skin tuberculosis of parrots and pigeons—nowadays a rare condition—is characterized by the development of sometimes stalked or keratinized skin growths in the facial region which may disintegrate at the base like tumors.

GIVING MEDICINES

The simplest way to administer medications is in dissolved form with the drinking water or mixed into the food. As the bird has a well-developed sense of taste, it will drink the water/drug mixture only reluctantly. In the end, however, thirst will be stronger than dislike. It goes without saying that all other water-filled containers—such as the bath—must be removed beforehand

1

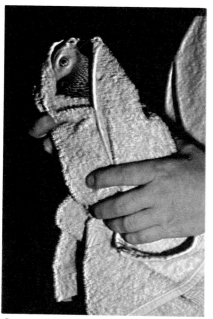

(1) A large bird such as this African grey parrot can be wrapped in a towel for handling, examination and maintenance of warmth during transport to a veterinarian. (2) The net used to capture a bird should be made of fine mesh so that the bird cannot become entangled and injure itself. (3) This budgerigar is being carefully removed from a net so that it can be examined.

2

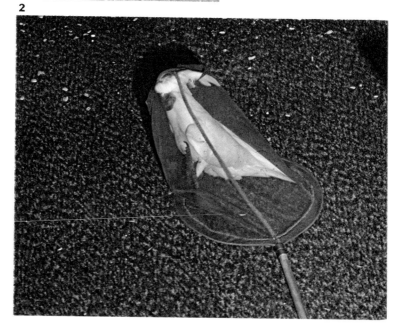

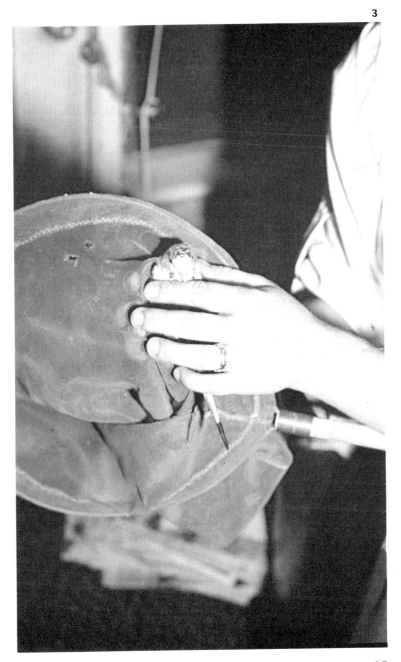

1

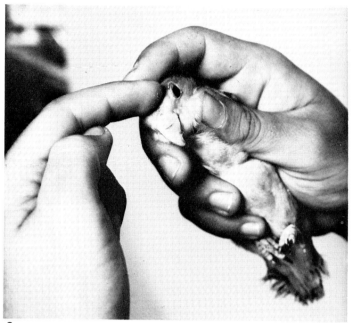

2

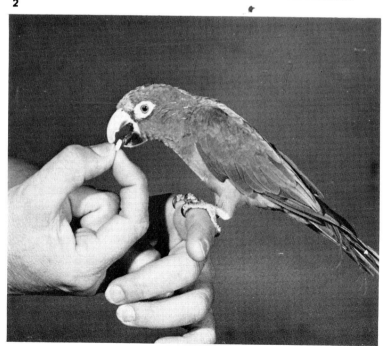

if the drinking water treatment is to succeed. Equally simple is the administration of a drug in aqueous solution or powder form if mixed into soft food. Seeds are moistened with the medication and subsequently ingested by the bird during husk removal.

On those rare occasions when a bird refuses water or food altogether, the drug is given by gentle force with the aid of a dropper. For this procedure the bird is held in the hand in such a way as to be sitting upright, for if it were to be force-fed the medication while lying in the hand, it might easily go the wrong way—the drug could get into the trachea and cause death by asphyxia. The bird only rarely opens the beak voluntarily—usually it is kept tightly closed. Where this happens we gently but firmly insert a sharpened matchstick, toothpick, or tweezer between the two halves of the beak. The drug can then be trickled into the opening by means of a pipette. The procedure is a similar one where sick and weakened birds need to be force-fed. Skilled bird keepers should be able to force-feed their charges without help from a second person.

A rather more unpleasant task is the administration of medicines to the great parrots who have an uncomfortably effective way of biting under such circumstances. These birds are best grabbed with a coarse cloth inside the cage, with the hands protected by thick leather gloves. A piece of wood is then placed between the bird's jaw so that it can bite into that, which is what usually happens, and the drug is gradually introduced from the side.

Medications can also be given to birds by injection, the site for this being the pectoral musculature. Wherever possible, however, this type of treatment should be left to the veterinarian.

(1) Should attempts like this to get the bird to open its beak fail, it will be necessary to pry it open with some object like a toothpick. (2) The owner of this halfmoon conure is lucky to have a bird that so willingly accepts medication.

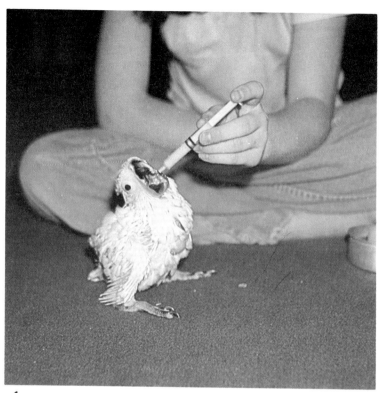

1

The same implements used to hand-feed baby birds are also suited to administering medication. (1) The plastic syringe employed to feed a young cockatoo will dispense accurate doses. Also, plastic and metal attachments for intubation are available from bird-supply houses. (2) A bent spoon may be used to force the beak open and then to trickle liquid down the bird's throat. (3) A plastic eyedropper is a quick and convenient dispenser for liquids.

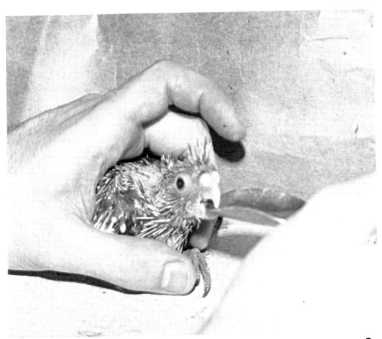

2

3

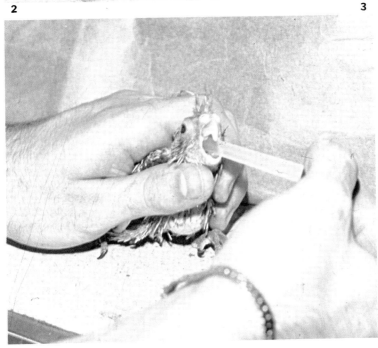

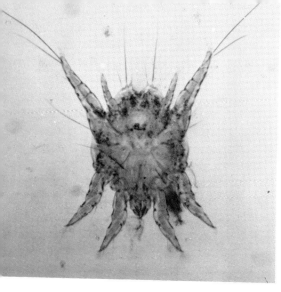

Left: Bird mite infestation may go so far as to produce a rash on the bird-keeper. **Below:** Prevention and control of mites is readily and safely accomplished by carefully following the directions for use of pesticides containing pyrethrins.

Diseases Caused By Parasites

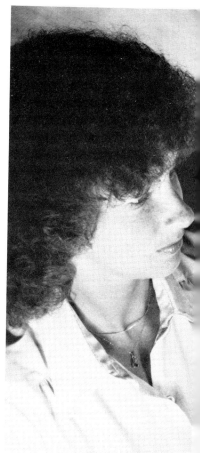

VIRUSES

Viruses are the smallest living things we know. They multiply only inside living cell tissue of the affected organism and are readily transmitted from one animal to another. Many viruses cause illnesses of epidemic proportions in animals and plants. Among the viral diseases of birds only psittacosis and pox are of significance to the keeper of small birds.

Bird Pox and Diphtheria

Causal agent: Bird pox is caused by the virus *Borreliota avium,* of which there are several varieties occuring as turkey, chicken,

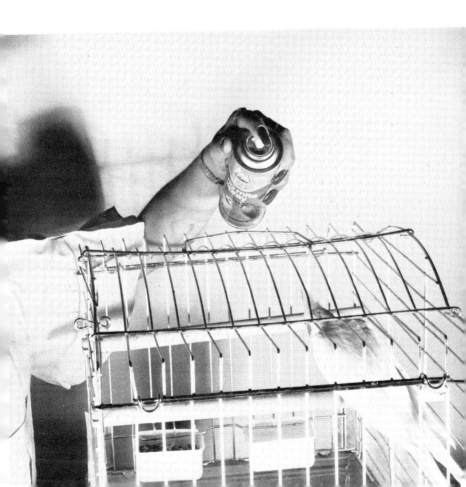

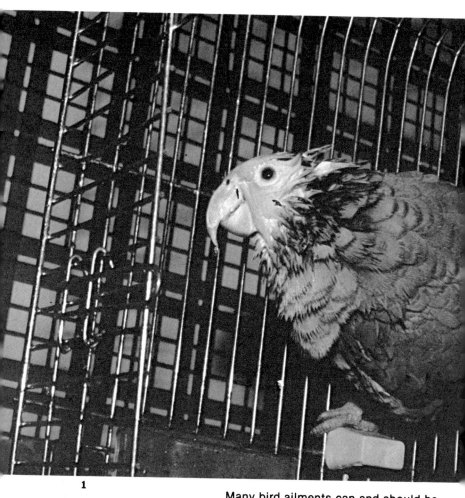

1

Many bird ailments can and should be prevented. (1) No bird, particularly after a bath, should be subjected to drafts or sudden changes in temperature. (2) All food and water provided for birds should be clean and fresh. Soft foods especially can become breeding grounds for disease-causing microorganisms.

2→

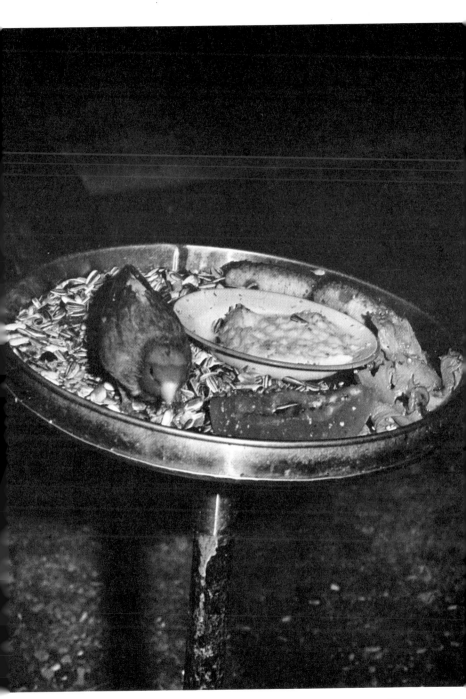

quail, pigeon, parrot, and canary pox respectively. Of the greatest importance to the bird keeper is canary pox.

Clinical picture and diagnosis: The course taken by this disease is extremely variable, as are the organic changes produced by it. It is hardly surprising, then, that such very different manifestations as skin pox (causing wart-like changes in the skin) and the deposit on the mucous membranes seen in diphtheria were once thought to be two independent diseases. It was not until relatively recently that research identified the pox virus as the common cause.

One form of bird pox, which expresses itself as septicemia or blood poisoning, runs a particularly rapid and malignant course, ending in the death of the affected bird just a few hours after infection. In cases like that the breeder is completely mystified at first.

More characteristic a course is run by the gasping-disease, which is well known and much dreaded in canary breeding circles. In this disease the victim develops a circulatory weakness causing severe shortage of breath. In the early stages of the illness the birds persistently shake their heads as though trying to get rid of something inside their beaks. Other affected individuals make squeaking and rattling noises when breathing and may have a short, dry cough. Shortly before the end, the sick bird tries to pump in the air through a wide-open beak. Eventually asphyxia sets in. The gasping-disease lasts for two to three days as a rule. Some birds suffer only minor symptoms of the disease, then make a quick recovery, and even manage to rear their young.

Where the pox runs a chronic course, yellowish nodules of pinhead size form at the edges of the beak, the eyelids, the pectoral region, and the epidermis of the wings, first becoming noticeable in the unfeathered areas of the skin. Later these nodules disintegrate on the surface and discharge a bloody fluid which coagulates to form dark brown scabs. On the eyelids one may sometimes see blister-like pustules with water contents. The conjunctiva may swell so severely that the whole eye is glued together.

Particularly in wild birds, we often find wart-like pox pustules on the toe joints which can assume considerable dimensions.

Subsequent obstruction of the blood vessels of the feet results in necrosis of the toe joints and foot.

The form of pox involving the mucous membranes, known as diphtheria, occurs on its own or in association with skin pox. It is characterized by white deposits on the mucous membranes of the oral cavity and throat which are either firmly attached or loosely distributed. When these adhering deposits are forcibly removed with tweezers or small sticks, copiously bleeding wounds result. Because of their thickness, the diphtheric deposits narrow the free nasal and oral cavity so severely that the bird can breathe and eat only with difficulty. Occasionally bits of scab become detached, are sucked into the trachea with the air, and get stuck in front of the fork that forms the two bronchi, killing the bird through asphyxia! Skin pox and diphtheric deposits sometimes persist for many weeks and then suddenly clear up.

Incidence and prognosis: Pox in passerine birds is particularly common among canary breeding stocks. The disease very often assumes epidemic proportions and wipes out entire stocks. The incidence and frequency of pox in our wild birds is not really known. Characteristic pox-type changes have been found in quail, doves, and many perching birds. The disease has also been identified in freshly imported Indian shamas, leaf birds, starlings, and flycatchers.

Acute forms of pox, among them the gasping-disease of canaries, cause high losses. Chronic forms, with skin pox and mucous deposits, frequently take a benign course, but long after their recovery the birds still excrete the pox virus and may infect newly purchased birds.

Treatment: In areas where the infection is common, breeders should avail themselves of the advantages of immunization. Some vaccines are manufactured from highly attenuated canary pox virus and give protection to the birds for a year (from about three weeks after immunization). Birds which are already infected cannot be cured by means of vaccination. In chronic cases, skin pox and mucous deposits may be painted with a solution of iodine and glycerine (1:2) once a day. This causes them to soften and makes it possible for them to be carefully removed with a small stick or a pair of tweezers the following day. Glued eyelids may be unstuck with the aid of boric acid solution (2%). A

(1) Spiralled claws are frequently a problem with finches, particularly of the genus *Lonchura* (nuns, or mannikins). (2) The dry gangrene of this canary's foot was caused by an overly tight band. In such cases, amputation is necessary. (3) Baldness (alopecia) in a canary. (4) The twisted neck (torticollis) and disorientation in this budgerigar may have its origin in either disease or vitamin deficiency.

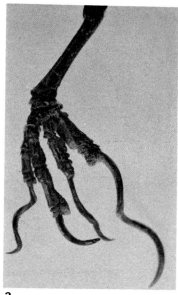

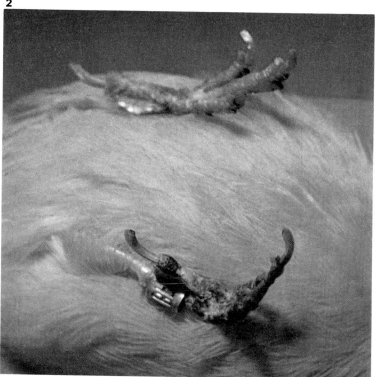

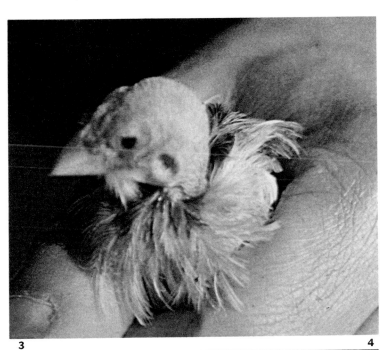

3

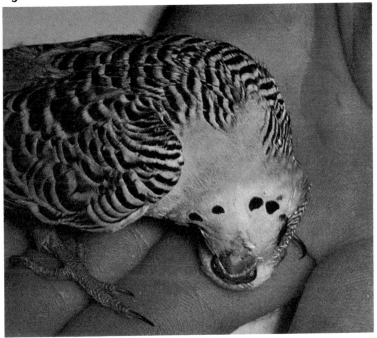

4

27

lyophilized canary vaccine has been produced. This vaccine, which is administered by intramuscular injection, has an excellent immunizing effect. It can also be used for emergency treatment of pox-infected stocks.

Fowl-pest

Causal agent: The virus of atypical fowl-pest.

Clinical picture and diagnosis: Parrots affected by fowl-pest exhibit twisting of the head, tremor, digital cramp, and paralysis. A proper identification of the disease can only be achieved by veterinarians.

Incidence and prognosis: Fowl-pest has long been known to occur in domestic hens and has also been diagnosed in a few other families. In 1970 in Holland and Germany, it was identified in parrots originating from South America and southern Asia, and it caused mass mortalities in quarantine stocks. Because the causal agent is readily transmitted to domestic hens, the importation of parrots from the above areas was prohibited. The few parrots who survive the disease are left with nerve damage which is almost always permanent. A cure is not possible.

BACTERIA

Bacteria are unicellular organisms belonging to a class of fission fungi (Schizomycetes) which can be seen only with the aid of a microscope. Only a few representatives of this vast group of microorganisms have become pathogens. Under favorable conditions they can multiply with extreme rapidity inside the animal body and be transmitted to other animals in saliva, urine, and feces. Of concern to the keeper of small birds are paratyphoid, pseudotuberculosis, and tuberculosis. An exact diagnosis of these diseases can only be made by a veterinarian.

Psittacosis

Causal agent: The microorganisms responsible for psittacosis is *Chlamydia psittaci,* which was once classified as a virus but today is regarded as a bacterium. Psittacosis and ornithosis are variants of the same causal agent. We speak of psittacosis when the disease occurs in parrots and of ornithosis when it affects birds of other species.

Clinical picture and diagnosis: Psittacosis does not produce typical symptoms in the bird. In severe infections there may be somnolence, diarrhea, nasal discharge, and pneumonia. The causal agent is frequently harbored and excreted by apparently healthy birds. The disease only breaks out when precipitated by unfavorable environmental conditions (transport, climatic changes, poor keeping conditions). Human beings generally get the disease through direct contact with the bird. One should never, therefore, allow a tame parrot to feed from one's mouth. In man the disease produces flu-like symptoms with headache, fever, and a slight cough; quite often the patient develops pleurisy. The disease lasts for about three to four weeks.

Incidence and prognosis: The disease is fairly common in imported parrots and may lie dormant in budgerigars. All species of birds can be affected, however. Few animal diseases are as well known to the general population and have sparked off such heated debates as psittacosis, which can be transmitted to man. Outbreaks in 1929/30 in 12 European countries resulted in a total of 800 people contracting the disease from imported parrots, and 143 people died. The import of parrots into Germany was banned in 1934 and it became compulsory to ring all parrots bred inside the country.

Similar outbreaks in the U.S. and other countries led to similarly restrictive measures. Successful treatment became possible with the discovery of antibiotics. Following their import, parrots (and most other birds) have to pass through a period of quarantine, during which time they are given antibiotics, often 5 mg of chlortetracycline (CTC) per gram of food per day. This dose is reached by adding 3 g of ready-mixed Aureomycin Chlortetracycline Mix 66 per 100 g of soft food, which may (for example) consist of rice, whole grain, and water (2:2:3). Budgerigars may receive 0.5 mg of CTC per gram of food per day for an uninterrupted period of 30 days. Where the disease breaks out in mixed populations of parrots and finches, all birds are treated. For sparrow-sized species, a CTC concentration of 0.5 mg per gram of food is sufficient where the above ready-mixed preparation is used. Treatment should last at least 30 days. The administration of antibiotics does not produce immunity to psittacosis.

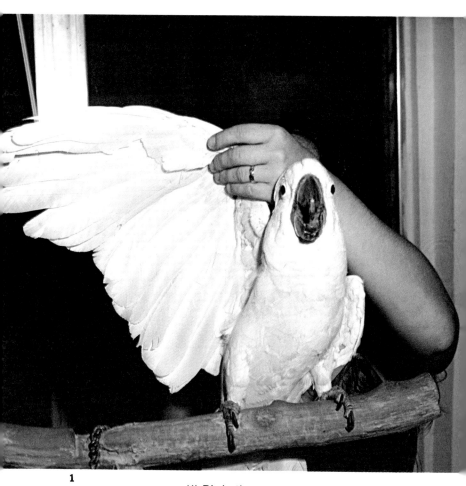

1

(1) Birds that appear restless or seem to be scratching themselves an inordinate amount of the time should be examined closely for mites and other parasites. (2) This budgerigar is suffering from a chronic case of scaly face, an infectious disease caused by a parasitizing mite of the genus *Cnemidocoptes.* Such "mange" mites live on their host on a permanent basis, burrowing into the upper layers of skin, laying eggs inside the tunnels so formed and feeding on skin substances and lymph.

2 →

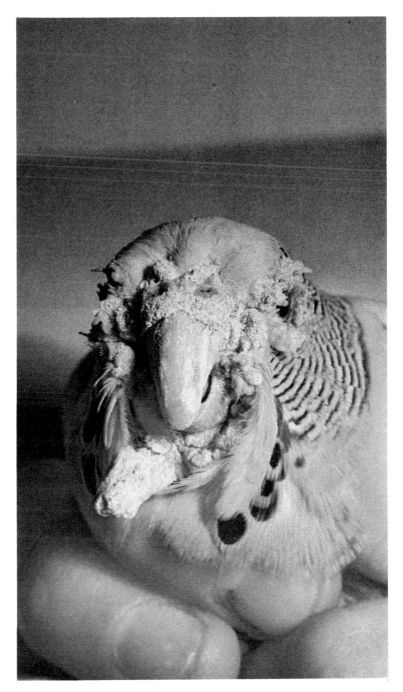

Paratyphoid

Causal agent: The disease is caused by bacteria of the paratyphoid group (genus *Salmonella*) which the bird ingests with infected food or water.

Clinical picture and diagnosis: Symptoms and the course of the disease in birds affected with paratyphoid depend on how resistant the body is and on the toxicity of the bacteria, which both vary a lot. If these germs are picked up by a bird weakened through transport or a chill, they can reproduce themselves in the body on such a vast scale that blood poisoning (septicemia) results, leading to the patient's death within hours. In such cases the bird falls dead from its perch without having shown very marked signs of disease beforehand.

In more resistant birds the disease manifests itself as a feverish illness. The animals sit on the perch trembling and fluffed-out; they sleep a lot and sift through the food without appetite. Diarrhea with slimy or watery feces hints at intestinal inflammation. Shortly before death there tends to be a circulatory weakness which makes the bird gasp for breath under rhythmical opening and shutting of the beak in a desperate way.

Where the disease runs a genuinely chronic course the bird, after having been off-color for weeks, develops swellings on the joints of the feet and wings. These result in lameness and inability to fly.

As the manifestations of paratyphoid are not very characteristic in the bird, a bacteriological investigation is needed for the diagnosis. Where the disease is suspected, a fecal specimen from the bird concerned should be tested by a veterinarian.

Incidence and prognosis: Among all the bacterial infections occurring in our cage and aviary birds, paratyphoid is the most common and has the highest mortality rate. The bird does not normally harbor such bacteria inside the body but picks them up when foraging for food in the vicinity of human settlements (in irrigated fields, for example). Healthy birds can carry paratyphoid germs without contracting the disease. For symptoms to develop, the birds need to be subjected to the kind of stress caused (for instance) by suddenly finding themselves in captivity: excitement, having to adapt to strange foods, tiring transport, and unhygienic accommodation in the dealer's cage. All these weaken the bird's resistance to such an extent that the bacteria can multiply with impunity and spread from the intestine to all other organs. Since a large stock of birds in a common cage almost always includes a few individuals which excrete these bacteria, the droppings of such carriers invariably infect food and drinking water before too long. An outbreak of the disease with high mortalities is the inevitable consequence.

Birds in aviaries have another dangerous source of infection to contend with: mice. These rodents very often harbor the germs and infect the birds' food with their feces and urine.

When early treatment is given, outbreaks of this disease can be brought under control within a short time.

Treatment: Antibiotics with a broad-spectrum action have proved successful in the treatment of paratyphoid. Particularly effective are chloramphenicol and the tetracyclines. These drugs are administered in high doses dissolved in the drinking water for a minimum of one week. After the course of treatment one should have the feces examined once more to make sure that the entire stock is in fact fully cured. Following treatment, cages and the indoor compartment of the aviary must be disinfected very thoroughly.

Pseudotuberculosis

Causal agent: This disease, in breeders' circles also known as paracholera and infectious necrosis of the canary, is caused by a bacterium, *Pasturella pseudotuberculosis rodentium.* The germs are generally picked up by the bird with food and drink contaminated by mouse droppings.

Clinical picture and diagnosis: These are just like a paratyphoid infection, so this disease also can run a short (acute) or a prolonged (chronic) course. The signs and symptoms observed in this condition do not differ from those of paratyphoid. The infection derives its name from the changes which develop in the internal organs and bear a strong resemblance to tuberculosis.

Incidence and prognosis: Pseudotuberculosis is less common than paratyphoid. The bacterium occurs inside the intestinal canal of healthy mice and rats, which appear to be the main reservoirs. Since the house mouse has a definite preference for living in seed shops and aviaries, an outbreak of this infection among one's bird population is a constant possibility. A diagnosis of pseudotuberculosis can only be made by dissection and bacteriological examination of a dead bird. If treatment is commenced early, the prognosis is favorable.

Treatment: For a cure of this disease, the same antibiotics as used in paratyphoid infection have proved effective. Since mice are the main carriers of pseudotuberculosis, rodent control is of special importance.

Tuberculosis

Causal agent: The bacillus occurring in birds is a special variant of tuberculosis. Avian tuberculosis affects all bird families, without exception. In parrots and canaries, human and bovine tuberculosis have also been identified.

Clinical picture and diagnosis: In birds, tuberculosis is a disease which progresses very slowly and can continue over many months. In the early weeks following infection, no signs of disease are noticed at all. Later the bird looks increasingly unwell, loses weight in spite of taking in food, does not come into molt, and in many cases suffers from diarrhea. In tubercular parrots and pigeons, skin proliferations may sometimes develop on the head. Outwardly these growths appear keratinized, but under their horny surface they show an ulcer-like disintegration. Since characteristic disease symptoms are absent, an exact determination of tuberculosis in the living bird is only possible with difficulty.

Incidence and prognosis: Where the keeping of small birds is concerned, tuberculosis is of virtually no significance nowadays. Until the turn of the century the disease frequently occurred in large parrots, which was directly linked to the high incidence of TB among the human population. Small wonder, then, that in those days it was virtually always the human TB bacillus that was isolated from affected parrots. Today, avian tuberculosis is from time to time introduced into the aviaries by infected mice, when it attacks above all terrestrial birds such as pheasants and quail. A cure for tubercular birds has not yet been found.

Treatment: Where cases of tuberculosis occur in a bird population, severe contamination of the aviary floor with tuberculosis bacilli must be expected. Since these bacteria are rapidly destroyed through dryness combined with ultraviolet rays (sunshine), the floor of the aviary is covered with sand or fine gravel and, wherever possible, all shade-forming plants are removed. For the effective disinfection of cages and of the indoor compartments of aviaries, Dekaseptol and carbolic acid (5%) are recommended. Most of the common disinfectants are ineffective against tuberculosis.

FUNGI
Aspergillosis

Causal agent: The most common cause of this disease is the mold *Aspergillus fumigatus*. Found almost everywhere in the world, this fungus forms a grayish green mold covering damp straw, hay, foodstuffs, rotting feces, and decaying wood. The spores of the fungus are released into the air with the slightest vibrations and remain airborne for a considerable time. While frequently inhaled by the bird, they only succeed in germinating on the mucous membranes of the respiratory tract if certain conditions prevail. A fungus infection only breaks out if the natural resistance of a captured bird has been seriously lowered by capture, changes in diet, and stressful transport.

Clinical picture and diagnosis: Mold growth on the bronchial mucosa, the lung tissue, and on the walls of the alveoli block the air passages and cause a shortage of breath. Under rhythmical opening and shutting of the beak the affected bird fights for breath until death is caused by asphyxia. Identical or similar difficulty in breathing also occurs in circulatory weakness, bronchial congestion, pneumonia, worm infestation of the trachea, and diphtheria.

Incidence and prognosis: Mold infections occur most frequently in newly imported tropical birds such as manikins, doves, trogons, tanagers, and turacos. The humid and sticky hothouse atmosphere which prevails in the jungle really ought to encourage the growth of mold, but frequent rainfall and the stillness of the air make it impossible for mold spores to become airborne among the trees. Thus the air remains "sterile." This explains, at least to some extent, why so many tropical birds have little resistance to aspergillosis.

Treatment: For a long time iodine glycerite was thought to be effective against the growth of mold fungi. Now, however, careful research has established the uselessness of this medium. Attempts to treat aspergillosis with new fungicidal agents such as Moronal (Mycostatin, Nystatin) and Flavofungin have proved disappointing. The reason for this lies in the late appearance of visible pathological changes. By the time labored respiration occurs the changes in the lungs and alveoli are so advanced that a cure has become impossible, even if the fungi are killed, because of severe and irreversible damage to the organs.

The main emphasis in the control of aspergillosis must, therefore, be placed on prevention. Newly imported species are particularly at risk and should be acclimated in clean, dust-free rooms. A well-balanced diet combined with vitamin therapy helps the bird to get through the dangerous phase of having to adapt to the unfamiliar environmental conditions of captivity more quickly. Once the body has regained its natural resistance the bird will be adequately protected against mold infections, too.

PROTOZA
Coccidiosis

Causal agent: Coccidians are microscopic unicellular organisms (belonging to the class Sporozoa) which occur in all species of birds in countless different varieties. In the majority of birds they parasitize the mucosal cells of the intestinal canal, there undergoing a complex developmental cycle of which phases of asexual reproduction (sporogeny) alternate with phases of sexual reproduction (merogony). Fertilization of the female cells (macrogametes) by the male cells (microgametes) is followed by the development of resistant forms (oocytes), roundish or oval formations with a thick membrane which are passed out in the bird's droppings. In damp soil they can remain infectious for weeks or months.

Although the wild bird, generally speaking, only ingests coccidian oocytes with its food in very small amounts, conditions are considerably more favorable for the disease in captivity. In densely stocked aviaries the resistant eggs excreted in the feces become so numerous that the bird picks them up in enormous quantities when feeding and drinking. The spores (sporozoites) released from the capsule inside the intestinal canal invade the mucosa of the gut and cause such severe injuries to it that a fatal intestinal inflammation is often the result.

Clinical picture and diagnosis: Manifestations of this disease in the bird are not very characteristic. The bird has a fluffed-up appearance, looks listless, and has no appetite. Almost always there is diarrhea that is slimy or bloody in character. In the final stages of the illness seizures and paralysis can sometimes be observed.

By means of the microscopic examination of a fecal specimen from the sick bird, coccidiosis can be diagnosed by the veterinary surgeon within a very short time.

Incidence and prognosis: Since most birds harbor individual coccidians in the intestine and excrete them in the feces, the resistant forms (oocytes) in the aviary soil rapidly increase in number. The damp, shady soil of well-planted aviaries and showcages extends the lifespan of the cysts considerably. Outbreaks of the disease with epidemic proportions are especially common among birds of over-stocked cages and aviaries, notably where the latter are not kept all that clean. The mass mortality of newly caught birds is invariably due to either coccidiosis or salmonellosis. If coccidiosis is identified in plenty of time, it should be possible for the stock to be saved.

Therapy: Coccidiosis can be treated successfully with sulfonamides. Among the many preparations available on the market, the following can be recommended as being well tolerated by small birds: Eleudron, Supronal, Socatyl, and Sulmet. The instructions for use enclosed with these sulfonamides should be followed as closely as possible since over-dosaging quickly results in poisoning of the birds. Preparations in an aqueous solution are administered with the drinking water or mixed into the soft food as powder.

To ensure that all the coccidians in the intestine – in their various forms and stages of development – are effectively obliterated, two courses of treatment are necessary. Ideally, the preparation concerned is given over a period of three to four consecutive days, followed by a three-day break, and then another three to four days of drug therapy. By this means the coccidians which left the intestinal mucosa and entered the gut after the first course of treatment are also destroyed. Since all sulfonamides deplete the body of vitamins, it is important to administer a multivitamin preparation in the drinking water when treatment has been completed.

To prevent reinfection with coccidian cysts, aviary birds should be placed in cages during treatment. The bottom of the hospital cage should be lined with paper which is changed several times a day. The top layer of the aviary soil, inevitably teeming with coccidian cysts, is removed (about one spade-cut deep) and replaced with healthy soil. Tests have shown that coccidian cysts in damp soil remain infectious to birds for up to 197 days.

Since most disinfectants are unable to penetrate the thick lipoid capsule of the cyst, it is best to use a 6% solution of Dekaseptol. When disinfecting a room, it is necessary to remove any obvious dirt with hot soda solution before applying the actual disinfectant.

WORMS
Tracheal worms

Causal agent: The bird disease known as "gape" is caused by the tracheal worm *Syngamus trachea*. It lives inside the trachea, adhering to the mucous membrane by suction, and feeds on the bird's blood (which gives the parasite a red color – "red worm"). The male of the species, attaining only 2 to 6 mm in length, is attached to the female's genital pore by the rear-end throughout its life, giving the impression of a two-headed creature. The female, which attains a maximum length of 2 mm, lays huge numbers of eggs. These reach the oral cavity with coughed-up slime, are generally swallowed, and find their way into the external environment via the digestive tract. In damp soil the larvae take one to two weeks to hatch. Together with soil they are frequently ingested by earthworms, slugs, and a variety of insects and remain alive inside their intermediate hosts for long periods, thus constituting a source of infection for birds. Encysted in the musculature of the earthworm, they were found to be still alive after more than four years. Inside the bird the tracheal worm has a lifespan of roughly four months.

Transmission to the bird takes place not only through the ingestion of infected food animals such as earthworms, slugs, or beetles, but also via food and water contaminated with infected droppings or mucus. Wild birds perching on the wire of the aviary drop their infected feces through it.

Clinical picture and diagnosis: Birds infested with tracheal worms cough, sneeze, yawn, and gasp for breath at frequent intervals, as well as attempting to rid themselves of sticky mucus by making thrusting movements with the head. When the windpipe is completely blocked by parasites and slime, the bird dies of suffocation.

Incidence and prognosis: Among the inhabitants of outdoor aviaries, gape is often very widespread during warm summers with a high rainfall since the eggs and larvae of the worms continue to be infectious for particularly long periods in wet soil. Whether a cure can be effected in small species of birds is doubtful.

Treatment: To date the destruction of tracheal worms remains difficult. Birds of starling- to raven-size may be treated with tincture of iodine diluted with water (9:1) or with Lugol's solution diluted with glycerine (1:5) and injected straight into the larynx with a curved cannula. The bird receives 0.1 ccm per day until cured. Barium antimonyl tartrate, used in the treatment of domestic chicks, can also be employed for birds of this size. The bird is placed inside a completely enclosed box and left to inhale the scattered powder. (Sparrow-sized species usually suffocate as a result of this method.) Another effective remedy for syngamosis is Thibenzole, an odorless and tasteless powder tolerated by small birds even when the dosage has been exceeded. Administer 10 mg of Thibenzole per 50 g of body weight over a period of one week. The drug can be stirred into the water or mixed into soft food.

Hair-worms

Causal agent: Hair-worms *(Capillaria)* occur in many species of birds. They usually live in the intestinal canal, though some species are found in the esophagus and the crop. The parasites attach themselves to the mucous membranes of these organs by suction and feed on the bird's blood. Infection takes place through ingestion of contaminated food, water, and soil. In years with a heavy rainfall the hair-worm brood in the damp soil of the aviary becomes so numerous that the bird population may suffer outbreaks of epidemic proportions.

Clinical picture and diagnosis: Heavy infestation with hairworms causes intestinal inflammation and thus diarrhea in the bird. There are no "characteristic symptoms," however.

Incidence and prognosis: Death through infestation with hairworms often sweeps through outdoor aviaries like an epidemic where budgerigars, pigeons, starlings, ravens, and domestic hens are concerned. If the disease is identified in good time (from fecal specimens or dead birds), treatment is successful.

Therapy: The only drug which is fully effective in the treatment of hair-worm infestation is Dekelmin (also available under the tradenames Promintic and Methyridine). Where a bird has been lost through hair-worm infestation, the whole population of the aviary concerned needs to be treated. For this purpose, the birds are put into cages and not given anything to drink from the afternoon of the day preceding treatment. On the following day, at about 10 A.M., Dekelmin dissolved in the drinking water is administered. To prevent cases of poisoning, the instructions for use must be closely adhered to.

To prevent reinfection, the infected soil of the aviary must be removed. Take off the top layer one spade-cut deep and replace with healthy soil.

Maw-worms

Causal agent: Maw-worms of the genus *Ascaridia* affect many families of birds, causing illnesses which can sometimes be fatal. Infection of the birds takes place through ingestion of worm eggs with contaminated soil, food, and water.

Clinical picture and diagnosis: Heavy infestation with mawworms in birds result in anemia and poisoning with the metabolic products excreted by the parasites. Large quantities of worms sometimes block the gut completely so that the bird dies of stoppage of the bowel. There are no characteristic manifestations in the bird.

Incidence and prognosis: Maw-worm infestation is common in parrots, pigeons, and fowl. Because these worms are strictly host-specific, pigeon maw-worms do not invade domestic hens and vice versa. Treatment of maw-worm infestation has a good chance of success.

Therapy: An effective preparation against maw-worms which is well tolerated by the bird is Piperazine. Since this drug kills only the maw-worms inside the intestinal lumen but not the larvae remaining in the tissue, treatment must be repeated six to eight weeks later. A dosage of 4 g piperazine phosphate to one liter of water has achieved good results in budgerigars with maw-worms.

Also remove the infected top layer of aviary soil to a depth of about one spade-cut and replace it with clean soil. As regards disinfecting the indoor areas of the aviary with firm flooring, the maw-worm eggs, having a very thick shell and hence being extremely resistant, can only be destroyed by means of a 6% Dekaseptol solution. Most other disinfectants are powerless.

Tapeworms

Causal agent: Although affecting all families of birds and large numbers of species, tapeworms only rarely cause disease symptoms in cage and aviary birds. Because these parasites have to pass through a complex developmental cycle via intermediate hosts before they become infectious to birds, they are soon gotten rid of again. If the intermediate host (an insect, worm, or snail) is absent, the developmental cycle of the tapeworm larva automatically comes to an end.

Clinical picture and diagnosis: Little is known about the detrimental effect of tapeworms on small birds. It is, however, unlikely that the damage is great. If on dissection of an emaciated bird severe tapeworm infestation is the only abnormality that can be found, then one is probably justified in taking these parasites to be the cause of death. Normally, however, a bird infected with tapeworms shows no signs of ill health, and the parasites are discovered purely by accident when tapeworm segments turn up in the bird's droppings.

Incidence and prognosis: Tapeworm infestation is fairly common in all newly imported wild birds, but it quickly clears up due to the lack of intermediate hosts. The sole exception to this rule seems to be the tapeworms of hummingbirds, where the fruit-fly *Drosophila,* which is an absolutely vital food animal, is thought to serve as intermediate host. This ensures the constant reinfection of these tiny birds. The expelling of tapeworms from the bird's body is possible.

Treatment: The most effective agent against tapeworms in the bird is Yomesan, which is marketed in tablet form. The tablets are dissolved in the bird's drinking water. Preparations containing Kamala and Arccoline were used a lot to control tapeworms in the past, but these drugs seem to have no real effect – while the segments of the tapeworm are shed, the head remains attached.

MITES
Red bird-mite

Causal agent: The red bird-mite *(Dermanyssus avium),* which grows to a size of 0.5 to 0.7 mm, prefers to stay in dark places and during the day hides away in cracks and crevices of cage and aviary corners. Popular hiding places are the grooves of perches, nesting baskets, and nesting materials of all kinds. By night the mites emerge to suck blood from the sleeping birds. In a severe infestation a few mites will usually be found on the bird's skin during the day as well, particularly under the wings. The female mite has a lifespan of eight weeks, during which it produces up to 2600 eggs. How soon the larvae hatch depends on the room temperature: at 9 to 10 °C, it takes five to eight days; at 19 to 20°C, 50 hours; and at 33 to 35°, a mere 36 hours. The period of maturation from larva to adult mite is seven days. The mite's color depends on its nutritional state: dark red mites have recently ingested blood, black ones have already digested the blood, and white or yellow ones are starving. Bird-mites can survive without nourishment for up to five months.

Clinical picture and diagnosis: Where the keeper notices that his birds are conspicuously restless on their perches at night, at short intervals nervously go through the feathers with the beak, and scratch themselves violently, mite infestation must usually be suspected. Unobservant keepers frequently do not detect these parasites until forced to experience the severe itching on their own skins – the red bird-mite briefly migrates to the human body as well, where it can cause a severe rash. In the bird, heavy infestation with mites results in advanced anemia and ultimately in death through exhaustion.

In spite of their small size, the mites are not too difficult to detect since they have a preference for certain hiding places. If, for example, the grooves on the perches are examined with a magnifying glass, mite eggs and feces in the form of gray and blackish deposits will be found. The parasites themselves, lively and agile, endeavor to escape from the light (which is unpleasant to them) into the darkness. One easy method of determining the presence of mites is to cover the cage with a white cotton cloth at night. The mites love to use this as their retreat, and in the morning they can be seen on it as red spots.

Incidence and prognosis: In birds kept in cages and aviaries, the red mite is the most common and most dangerous ectoparasite (external parasite). In pet shops with their heavy turnover of stock, mite infestation is fairly common, too, and when new birds are bought the parasites are all too easily introduced into mite-free stocks. Since the bird-mites multiply very rapidly, they become established and widely distributed within a short time. With the help of an insecticide the destruction of the mites presents no insurmountable difficulties. A weakened bird whose appetite is not impaired by the constant blood-loss quickly recovers if given plenty of nourishing food.

Control: Once the keeper has discovered that his birds are infested with mites, treatment should commence without delay (for the birds' sake, if nothing else!). The contact insecticides which are now used for the destruction of mites are not without danger to the bird and should be handled with great caution. Prior to application the birds should be taken out of the aviary and put into a mite-free cage which is transferred to another room. Cage birds are moved into another mite-free cage. The empty cages and aviaries are sprayed thoroughly with an insecticide in aqueous solution. Nesting places and perches must not be forgotten, and nesting material is burned. If one wants to make absolutely sure, the insecticide can be left to act for several days. Afterwards the rooms are intensively aired and the water and seed cups washed. Only then can the birds be moved back. Where small metal cages are involved, it is usually sufficient to rinse them in boiling water. The cage and the surrounding area are also sprayed with an insecticide. It must be remembered that the mites like to sit under loose wallpaper as well and in cracks in the wall.

To kill off individual mites sitting in the bird's plumage, the feathers are treated with a powdered insecticide. When doing this the keeper should carefully protect the bird's head with his hand to prevent the animal from breathing in the preparation. The safety precautions emphasized here regarding the application of insecticides may seem exaggerated, but many birds have actually been damaged or even killed by preparations sold as "guaranteed harmless." Consult your veterinarian as to the best insecticide to use on your birds.

Scaly Face

Clinical picture and diagnosis: This disease of budgerigars is caused by the mite *Cnemidocoptes pilae.* The first changes due to this form of mange usually appear at the side of the beak in the form of a barely visible grayish white deposit. Weeks or months later, crusty deposits can be seen in this area, which now looks as though it were sprinkled with flour. These foci gradually spread to the surrounding skin. Such scabs are proliferating horny substances which have developed as a result of chronic skin inflammations caused by the mites.

From the angle of the beak the condition spreads to the beak itself and to the cere and the skin of the eyelids. In cases of severe mite infestation the entire facial region may be covered with crusty deposits, and often these changes also spread to the chin, the cloacal region, and the legs. However, while the head is always affected and is always the first part to be involved, the other areas of the body just mentioned are affected irregularly or not at all.

The ceaseless burrowing activity of the mange mites lends a spongy, porous look to the skin scabs or crusts, the horny part of the beak, and the ceres which is highly characteristic of this disease. The chronic inflammation of the horny part of the beak leads to uninhibited growth of the latter and thus to the formation of abnormally long and crossed beaks.

Some of the skin changes seen in scaly face may be confused with other diseases. Small nodules which form on the skin of the eyelids resemble pox. The floury white deposit and the porous consistency of the new growth, however, point toward mange. Where long, stalked horny growths appear on the eyelids, one may be reminded of tuberculosis of the skin. Tubercular skin changes also lack the spongy, porous consistency, however.

Incidence and prognosis: Scaly face is common among budgerigar populations, but in the early stages it tends to escape notice. The disease primarily affects birds of three months to two years of age. Years may elapse between initial infection and the outbreak of mange. A four-year-old budgerigar which had not come in contact with members of its species for 3½ years suddenly suffered from scaly face. It would appear that the mites cannot multiply to any great extent until the bird's resistance has been seriously lowered by molt problems, colds, and other adverse factors. After experimental transmission of mange mites to two budgerigars, the first—which suffered from chronic intestinal inflammation—showed scabs at the sides of the beak after just 14 days. The second bird—a strong and very healthy specimen—still did not present any changes even after two months. To generalize, scaly face has a preference for bird populations kept in an unfavorable environment, such as in dark, damp cellars. The prognosis is good where this illness is concerned.

Treatment: Various preparations have proved effective in mange. They are brushed on in liquid form. When applying them, however, not only the visibly changed areas of the skin should be treated, but also all those areas which are known to be favored by mites although not yet showing any abnormalities. In other words, the preparation is painted onto the whole area around the beak, the eyelids, the cloacal region, and the legs. Odylen, a sulfur compound, is applied undiluted at intervals of two to three days, and any scabs that have become detached are carefully removed. To effect a cure, four applications are generally sufficient as a rule. To be on the safe side, however, it is recommended to repeat the treatment two to three weeks later.

I must point out here that other drugs have a highly toxic effect, and even Odylen can sometimes prove lethal in delicate species of small birds, for example Gouldian finches, especially where already weakened animals are involved. Treatment of mangy areas of the skin with ordinary mineral oil (recommended on account of its safety), with the view of blocking the respiratory pores (tracheae) of the mites, has not brought general success.

Foot mange of perching birds

Causal agent: This disease is caused by the mange mite *Cnemidocoptes jamaicensis,* which infects almost exclusively the feet.

Clinical picture and diagnosis: The boring and burrowing activities of the mites in the horny plates of the foot and toes first of all result in the formation of scales. Later, crusty, furrowed deposits form which look as though dusted with flour. The considerable thickening of the feet seriously impedes the bird's movement, and the constant itchiness causes severe irritation.

Incidence and prognosis: Foot mange occurs in all passerines, although it is most frequently seen in canaries and sparrows. The chances of a complete recovery are good.

Therapy: Treatment is the same as for scaly face.

Foot mange of game birds

Causal agent: The cause of the disease is the mange mite *Cnemidocoptes mutans,* which affects fowl and game birds. It attacks only the legs. The changes caused by this mite are thickened legs and feet.

Clinical picture and diagnosis: The chronic inflammation resulting from the burrowing activity of the mange mite in the hypodermis of the legs and feet leads to proliferations of the horny substance. Underneath the horny plates a dry, chalky gray deposit forms which raises the plates and eventually gives a shapeless appearance to the leg ("elephant's foot"). Thickening of the foot makes movement increasingly difficult, thus indirectly causing starvation, emaciation, and ultimately death.

Incidence and prognosis: Foot mange in the aviary occasionally occurs in small gamebirds such as quail, partridge, rock fowl, and francolin. The prognosis is good.

Treatment: This is the same as for scaly face.

BIRD-LICE

Causal agent: Bird-lice (Mallophaga) are common skin

parasites of birds. These brown, wingless insects which attain a length of 1 to 3 mm move about very actively among the bird's feathers and feed mainly on scales and feather particles. They attach their egg parcels to the base of the feather quills in the down feather area.

Identification: By crawling about on the feathers and the skin, the bird-lice cause an intense itchiness, making the bird bite and scratch itself frequently.

Incidence and prognosis: Bird-lice occur in all birds that have been freshly caught. If detected in large numbers on a bird that has already been living in captivity for some time, then this usually indicates that the animal is suffering from some kind of internal disease. The healthy bird generally harbors only few of these parasites. The prognosis is favorable.

Therapy: The bird is dusted with an insecticide powder. For this purpose, the bird is picked up with the hand and, while receiving treatment, has its eyes and nostrils protected by a cloth or paper collar. Treatment should be repeated several times at intervals of ten days to ensure that any lice that have newly hatched are also destroyed.

NEST PARASITES

The nests of birds are common breeding grounds for many parasites such as bird-bugs, fleas, ticks, mites, biting flies, and the maggots of flies. Flies of the genera *Lucila, Protocalliphora, Chrysoma,* and others like to lay their eggs in tiny skin wounds and the ears of naked nestlings. The hatched larvae soften the surrounding tissue with their secretions. As a result, the bird develops ulcers and inflammations which are often fatal. Nestlings are not infrequently eaten alive by maggots.

If the keeper finds affected young birds in his own nests, he is advised to burn the nesting material. If for any reason he wants to go on using it for rearing purposes, it should be dusted very thoroughly with an insecticide powder such as Pyrethrum. Any ticks, fleas, and biting flies attached to the chicks are carefully removed with pointed tweezers. Wounds caused by these insects are disinfected with quinoline or potassium permanganate solution.

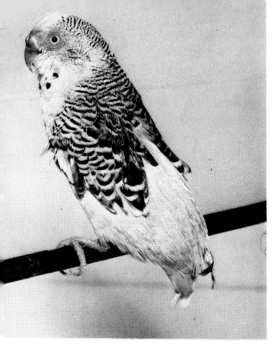

Left: This five-year-old male budgerigar has lost his tail and flight feathers due to French molt. **Below:** Pet shops carry a wide range of products especially designed to make the job of caring for birds easier.

Problems
of
the
Skin
and
Appendages

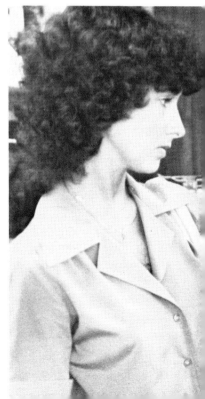

SKIN TEARS

Injuries of the skin are most commonly seen on the head. They are generally contracted during fights with members of the same species. The rest of the body occasionally suffers lacerations and stabbing wounds caused in nocturnal agitation through flying against sharp objects such as nails projecting from the wall, sharp ends of wire, and wooden splinters on the wall of the aviary. Birds which spend the night clinging to the wire of the aviary may be injured by the sharp claws of cats and owls.

Generally speaking, the bird's skin possesses excellent natural healing powers which make treatment superfluous where many minor injuries to the skin are concerned. Where the head has been injured so severely, however, that entire folds of skin hang down in patches, these must be reunited with tweezers and a few stitches put in. For disinfection an antiseptic powder is used. If the bird scrapes or scratches at the sutured wound, as frequently

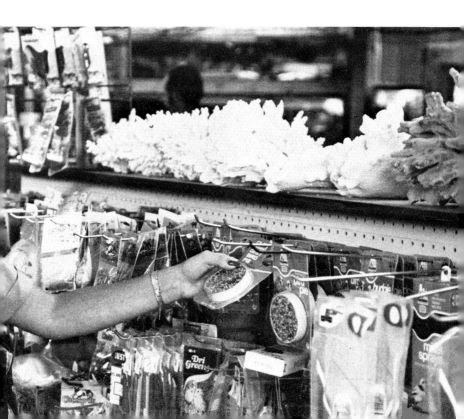

happens with parrots, a collar of the appropriate size should be fitted. The edges of the wound completely rejoin within just a few days. If head injuries of this nature are left untreated, the bird will be marked with a bald patch for the rest of its life. Larger lacerations to the body, which are not very common, must be sutured, too. To minimize blood-loss which in small birds rapidly causes weakness, coagulant powder should always be kept handy. To prevent other birds from pecking at the wounds, the patient is kept in isolation.

Bald patches on the back of the head and on the neck in female pigeons and quail are frequently produced during the act of mating when the cock pushes his beak into the female's feathers in these areas. Lost feathers are soon replaced once the pair have been separated. Painting the bald skin patches with an alcoholic solution of Peruvian balsam speeds up the growth of new feathers.

In weaver finches (though not exclusively) one frequently observes baldness (alopecia). Among the waxbills kept in cages it is very common in strawberry finches, golden-breasted waxbills, red-tailed lavender finches, and violet-eared waxbills, while being extremely rare in black-rumped waxbills, orange-cheeked waxbills, and other species. Keepers differ in their opinions as to the cause of such bald patches. Mutual plucking, vitamin A deficiency, and too dark a cage locality have all been blamed. In the majority of cases, if the "baldies" are exposed to the fresh air in an outdoor aviary the naked skin patches will soon be covered with feathers again.

Abnormal Growth of the Beak and Claws

In caged seed-eaters and more rarely in insectivores, one occasionally observes beaks that have grown abnormally long, crooked, or crossed. Abnormal length of one or both tips of the beak in cage birds is caused by insufficient wear and tear of the horn and by faulty nutrition. Among the northern finches it is above all the goldfinch which suffers from beak abnormalities, because in captivity it cannot rub the horn on thistle heads as it does in nature. An abnormally long upper tip of the beak is frequently seen in insectivores. The protruding part periodically breaks off by itself, however (beak molt).

In the budgerigar the upper beak sometimes grows so far down in a strong curve that its tip touches the crop area and injures the skin by rubbing against it. The same malformation of the beak can also be seen in scaly face. In that case, however, the greatly extended upper beak is of a pumice-like porous consistency due to the tunnelling of the mites.

Crooked and crossed beaks can affect all species of birds, although they are more common only in budgerigars. According to breeders, abnormal growth of the beak may develop in the nestling due to a crooked-billed or cross-billed parent bird twisting the as yet very soft and pliable beaks of the young when feeding them. It is much more likely, however, that such malformations in the budgerigar are hereditary, for similar abnormalities also occur as mutations in domestic fowl from time to time and have been observed in wild birds on more than one occasion.

A bird with a malformed beak is often unable to take enough food, so it consequently suffers a progressive weight-loss. It will die of starvation if the keeper does not make a timely decision in favor of treatment.

To trim the abnormally long mandible, hold the bird's head between the thumb and index finger. Then, using scissors or a sharp knife, cut back the projecting horny substance to its normal length and rub away any sharp edges with fine sandpaper. Brittle horn tends to splinter and should therefore be brushed with warm glycerine, olive oil, or mineral oil prior to being clipped.

In cases of crossed mandibles it is usually necessary to repeat the operation at intervals of several weeks since the horn cannot wear down "automatically" owing to the abnormal position of the mandibles to each other. If during the operation blood oozes from the cut area, this can be arrested by applying coagulant powder.

The keeper can prevent many beak abnormalities by providing cuttlebone, calcium blocks, and grit. When the bird goes to work on these hard materials the horny parts of the beak are worn down just as they are in nature. In insectivores with abnormally long or crossed beaks or with the mandibles growing sideways, a cure can sometimes be effected by administering vitamin A.

Abnormal growth of the claws is a side effect of cage-dwelling and can thus occur in all cage birds. Due to insufficient wear and tear, the horny claws grow in length, not infrequently assuming a spiral shape. This kind of abnormality of the claws is almost the rule in weavers and waxbills.

To trim the claws, hold the bird in your hand and fix the foot to be treated between your ring finger and little finger. When cutting the claws it is important not to injure the blood vessels which reach far into the horny parts of the foot. The course of the blood vessels is clearly visible in the light horny substance. In many cases, unfortunately, the blood vessel extends with the proliferating claws so that cutting it cannot be avoided. The resultant bleeding is not dangerous and can be arrested with coagulant powder.

Molt

Molt in the bird is understood to mean renewal of the feathers. Molting takes place at regular intervals and is a vital process since the feathers suffer considerable wear and tear during the course of the year. At what time of the year the bird molts depends on the species. Thus most northern song birds replace their entire plumage shortly before the migratory period in late summer. Others may molt twice a year, a complete molt in the summer and a partial one (of the small feathers only) in their tropical winter quarters. Still others molt only once, in their winter home. The process of feather replacement is particularly obvious in certain species such as (male) weaver finches and whydah birds, which exchange their inconspicuous grayish brown "resting plumage" for colorful breeding plumage.

Older wild birds frequently molt only with difficulty or not at all in their first year of captivity, since the change in nutrition the organism is subjected to causes considerable problems. In healthy and acclimated birds, on the other hand, the molt proceeds without complications. A prolonged, interrupted molt, let alone an absence of molting, is therefore a serious indicator of a weakened organism.

Molting difficulties have many causes, although in most cases of that nature faulty nutrition will be the main culprit. A bird which is under-exercised, since it lives in a confined space yet receives a diet with far too great a calorie content or is getting a monotonous and vitamin-deficient diet or food which is difficult to digest, is not in a position to undergo a normal molt. Where a bird has difficulties in molting or will not molt at all, feather replacement can be stimulated by various methods. By providing insectivores and many seed-eaters with fresh animal protein in the form of live ant pupae, fly maggots, and insects, it is often possible to induce molting. Another useful stimulant of the metabolism is a daily bath; birds which are not keen on entering the bath are sprayed with tepid water each day. Several half-hour sessions per day of infra-red radiation intensify the metabolic activites and, even in delicate insectivores, often produce the onset of molting. The value of mixing fresh thyroid gland or thyroid preparations into the food is still being debated. In some species an abrupt molt results, while in others there is no reaction at all.

Tail or wing feathers which are excessively worn or have broken off can be pulled out by the keeper (this is done very quickly). They should not, however, all be removed at once, but must be pulled individually or, at most, in pairs at intervals of three to four days. The new feathers grow within 14 days.

If molting has already begun but comes to a sudden halt, the interruption may be due to a drastic change in temperature or be caused by a chill through drafts or a sudden dietary change. The keeper must always bear in mind that a molting bird needs to be looked after with particular care!

French Molt in the Budgerigar

French molt is a disease of the feathers occurring in very young budgerigars which are just beginning to fly. The disease is widespread in budgerigar populations and causes breeders a lot of worry. Shortly before or after leaving the nesting box, the young birds suddenly, without any apparent reason, lose their flight feathers, tail feathers, and sometimes part of their body feathers as well. The shed feathers clearly show a narrowing of the quill a few centimeters above the root. The young budgerigars run about on the bottom of the cage unable to fly, hence they are referred to as "runners" or "creepers." If they are well developed, the lost feathers will grow again within eight to ten weeks, and from then on it will be impossible to tell the former runners from the healthy birds.

The name "French molt" was given to the disease because it frequently afflicted the descendants of budgerigars that had been imported into Germany from France. It is not a degenerative condition acquired in captivity but has repeatedly been observed among wild parrots in Australia as well, where the affected young, unable to fly, fall prey to their numerous predators. In their search for the cause of the disease, breeders have variously put the blame on feather mites, high nesting box temperatures, faulty feeding, and bacteria.

Breeding experiments carried out by scientists in order to track down the cause of the runner problem established that what we are concerned with here is a genetic disease triggered off by a single hereditary factor with incomplete dominance. There seem to be other precipitating factors as well, however. Thus Enehjelm transferred young birds originating from runner-producing parents to the care of normal pairs and received normal young, but runners still developed when the young were transferred at 11 to 12 days of age. Enehjelm concludes from this that there exists a critical period for young which are fed by runner parents, somewhere during the first ten days of life. The cause of this phenomenon seems to lie in protein-deficient crop milk of the runner parents, and this too has been proved experimentally. The inability of certain budgerigars to produce high-protein crop milk could also depend on hereditary factors. This would make the tendency of some pairs to breed runners an indirectly hereditary condition.

Until the problem sees a final solution, it is recommended that the breeding pairs be provided with the best possible living conditions, are not over-bred (*i.e.,* forced to produce more than two clutches per year with three to four young each), and that a raising-food with a high protein and vitamin content be used. Weakly and degenerative birds should always be destroyed, and "runners" should only exceptionally be used for breeding. On the other hand, valuable breeding pairs that have occasionally produced individual runners should not be immediately exterminated, although for practical reasons this is hardly possible.

54

Feather-Plucking in Parrots

A common phenomenon among caged parrots is feather-plucking or feather-eating, which soon causes a greater or lesser degree of baldness in the affected birds. While it used to be generally thought that lack of stimulation and exercise was responsible for this "vice" in the parrots, U. Schmitt recently pointed toward another cause. When his macaw suddenly became a feather-plucker, Schmitt tried all the remedies that had so far been recommended. Yet vitamin therapy, the application of sprays with bitter substances, and the acquisition of other macaws to prevent boredom brought no improvement. After observing that macaws in a zoo, although living in poor conditions, had healthy plumages and were fed with all sorts of salty snacks by the public, he experimentally gave his three (by now!) feather-plucking macaws a good pinch of salt in a half liter of water every day. One macaw immediately stopped the feather-plucking, while a second continued for a few more months, and the third continued for as long as a whole year. Thereafter all three macaws had a perfect plumage. Considering that free-living parrots often take in salty soil and budgerigars enjoy picking up salt grains from the bottom of the cage, it is probably safe to assume that at least in a proportion of feather-pluckers the habit is caused by salt deficiency. These birds simply obtain the necessary quantity of salt which is absent from their diet by chewing fresh feather quills. Such a feather-plucking parrot is, therefore, given a generous pinch of salt in a half liter of water per day, this in a separate cup in addition to its normal drinking water. The salt must not be sprinkled over the food, as this could cause poisoning. Schmitt observed that a bird only drinks as much salty water as it can tolerate without ill effects. He stressed that a former feather-plucker may have to be treated by this means for the rest of its life to prevent relapse. Since the daily administration of salt water is neither time-consuming nor costly, it is a "luxury" every parrot owner can afford. You must be patient, however, in case the desired success is not achieved instantly.

Rarely, a parrot loses all its feathers without having plucked them. Here the cause is suspected to be a disturbance of the endocrine glands. A cure is not known.

FRACTURES

Fractures of the bones of the feet, legs, toes, and wings are far from rare in birds and generally result from flying into obstacles or becoming entangled in wires. If one is known to be a bird fancier, people quite often come along with birds that have sustained those types of injuries. Generally speaking, fractures in the bird heal without any problem and much more quickly than in humans - within as little as 10 to 14 days the fractured bones have knitted together again sufficiently for the limbs concerned to be used. The rapid regeneration of the bone tissue is presumably due to the bird's high metabolic rate.

Fractures of the bones of the leg

In the wild bird, fractures of the bones of the leg usually heal so well that the affected limb becomes fully functional again. That the ends of the fracture frequently grow together in some crooked way is of little consequence to the bird's ability to survive. In the case of fractured upper and lower thigh bones, a splint cannot be applied because of their anatomical position, and in fractures of the toe joints a splint is unnecessary since they heal very quickly without any kind of treatment. A splint is called for only in fractures of the foot. Here the chances of healing depend on the condition of the fractured area. If the broken end of the bone is attached by nothing more than a few bits of skin and ligament, a recovery can no longer be expected and the leg must be amputated. On the other hand, there are good grounds for optimism where the upper end of the foot has merely been bent over the lower one and muscles, blood vessels, and ligaments have not been torn.

To apply a splint to a fractured lower leg bone, the bird is held in the hand belly-up. The fractured surfaces are pressed together in such a way that the leg bone regains its natural position and the splint is fitted to extend upward from the base of the toes to just below the leg joint. The material used for the splint may be anything from feather quills, straws, and toothpicks to matches and similar items. The lower leg bone and splint are then kept in position with woollen thread, tape, or elastoplast, and on top of that a layer of collodion or plaster of Paris. When the bandage is to be removed the glues can be readily dissolved with ether or acetone. The bandage may be taken off after 14 days.

Fractures of the Wings

Fractures of the bones of the wings are almost always sustained by flying into hard surfaces and objects such as glass panes and thin wires. Since the bird often achieves high flight speeds, the force of the impact is quite considerable, frequently leading to cerebral concussion as well. The bones of the wing are thin, light, and brittle owing to a high calcium content and are partially filled with air, so they break into a lot of fragments. This makes it very difficult for the fractured surfaces to grow together again in such a way that function is restored. A further complication is that if even a small strand of muscle fiber is damaged, there may be disturbances in the rhythm of movement of the flight muscles and then it is doubtful whether the bird will ever be able to fly properly again. As opposed to a leg fracture, a fractured wing in a wild bird means certain death.

Splints are not used in fractures of the wings. One merely puts the drooping wing back into its natural position and straps it firmly to the body with a muslin bandage. To ensure that the bandage is securely in place, it must be passed across the back and over both wings and then crossed between the legs. To prevent severe friction on the wings, since these have been pressed against the lateral wall of the chest, they are padded with cotton. Parrots which constantly chew on their bandages can be a nuisance. These birds have to be provided with collars of celluloid or some other plastic. Needless to say, they do not feel comfortable with this foreign body around the neck, but generally they get used to it after a while. Fractured wings commonly take as long as 21 days to heal. When the bandage is taken off the wing still hangs down slightly in most cases, but it will soon return to its natural position. Unfortunately, however, birds with healed fractures of the wing seldom regain their full powers of flight and can only be kept alive in human care.

Birds with bandages on legs or wings should be given a small hospital cage with a soft, well-cushioned bottom layer and low perches.

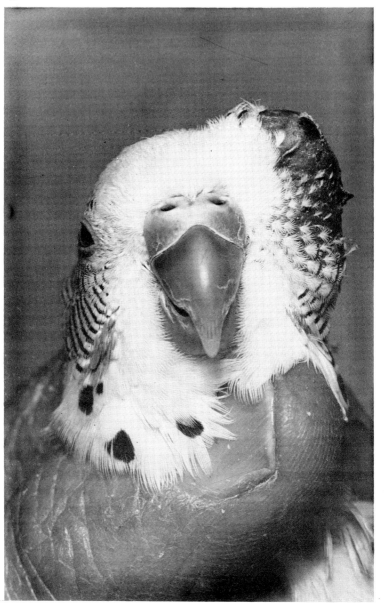

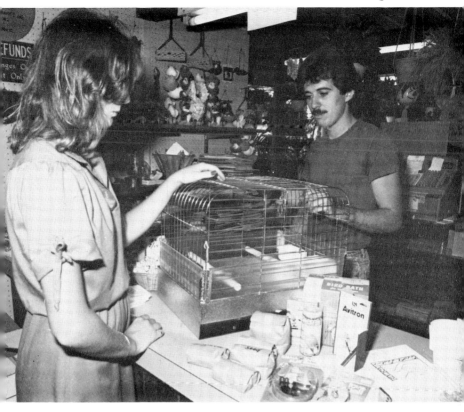

(1) When you purchase a cage, make sure that the cage is the proper size for the bird you plan to house in it. It should be large enough that the bird can exercise. (2) Long before any swelling becomes as extensive as shown here a veterinarian should be consulted.

Amputation

If a bird has suffered a compound fracture and there is no chance of a recovery, the broken limb will need to be amputated. To prevent copious bleeding, a tight bandage is applied to the limb just above the amputation site. Then the fractured limb is quickly cut off with scissors. Antibiotic and coagulant powders should be kept in readiness for operations of this nature. The caged bird soon gets used to the loss of a foot or wing and suffers little as a result.

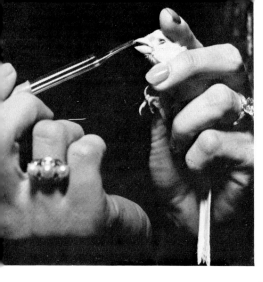

Left: This is the proper way to use an eyedropper to administer medication to a small bird: be sure the bird is held vertically. **Below:** Whenever you use one of the many bird products available at pet shops, be sure to carefully follow the directions given on the container.

*Diseases
of
the
Internal
Organs*

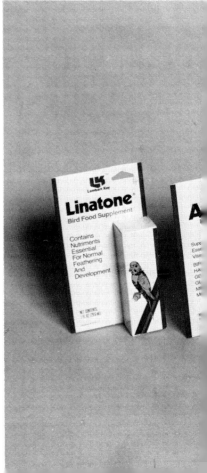

THE DIGESTIVE SYSTEM
Structure of the Alimentary Canal

In many species of birds the esophagus expands into a pouch-like chamber (the crop) just before it enters the chest. The crop has the function of softening and steeping the food. Pigeons possess two symmetrical crops lined with mucous membrane which produces a fatty white substance, crop milk, during the breeding season. This "milk" is the product of fatty transformation of the crop mucosa and contributes to the nutrition of the young.

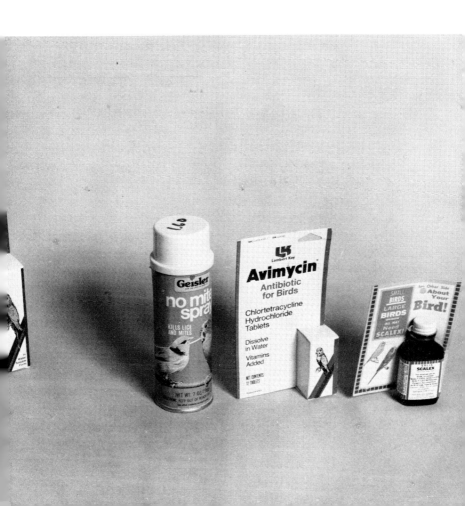

From the crop the food passes into the glandular part of the stomach where it is partially digested by protein-splitting pepsin in the presence of hydrochloric acid. It then moves on to the muscular part of the stomach, the gizzard, where it is eventually ground down by the combined action of muscular movement and grit or small stones. The thickness of the gizzard wall varies with the dietary adaptations of the species. Thus seed-eaters have a strong gizzard musculature while meat- and fish-eating birds possess nothing more than a thin elastic gastric sac.

The intestinal canal of birds is characterized by possessing two blind tubes (ceca) which vary in length from family to family, in some being nothing more than small sacs. The end of the intestine widens into the sac-like cloaca and also receives the ureters and the sperm ducts or the oviducts.

Crop Binding

Cause: Crop binding usually develops as a result of the too hasty ingestion of large quantities of seeds. If the bird drinks water afterwards, the seeds swell inside the crop, stretching the crop walls so severely that the musculature is unable to pass the wedged contents on to the stomach; eventually the muscles grow flaccid. In fowl, crop binding can also be caused by the swallowing of long grass blades which conglomerate into balls inside the crop.

Clinical picture and diagnosis: The crop is overly full and thus clearly visible as a semispherical bulge. It feels doughy or hard to the touch. The bird is not as lively as usual, and from time to time it opens the beak as though yawning. If the build-up of food presses against the trachea, the condition may lead to difficulty in breathing; such birds anxiously keep their beaks down.

Incidence and prognosis: In cage and aviary birds, crop binding is a rare disease. The chances of a cure are good, provided treatment is commenced early.

Therapy: By gentle massage of the crop with thumb and index finger, one seeks to induce the accumulation of food to move in the direction of the beak. In many cases – and whenever matted plant substances are the cause – only an incision into the crop can bring relief. Since wounds in the bird have a tendency to heal quickly, the incision will soon close up again. Nevertheless, it is preferable to leave this operation to the veterinary surgeon for the simple reason that in certain species of birds (pigeons, for example) the crop wall is so vascular that copious bleeding results.

Crop Congestion

Cause: How crop congestion develops in small birds remains largely a mystery. Infectious crop inflammations have been described in finches and budgerigars, but a specific cause still needs to be found.

Clinical picture and diagnosis: The bird shows a diminished appetite, frequently stretches the neck, makes drinking or swallowing movements, and shakes its head from time to time, flinging an evil-smelling fluid from the beak and nostrils. The crop itself may be severely distended through the presence of putrid gases. On dissection the crop is found to contain small quantities of a stinking liquid with foam or bubbles on the top.

In the budgerigar a diphtheroid crop inflammation occurs, characterized by the formation of thick yellowish deposits on the crop mucosa and the lower regions of the esophagus which obstruct the passage of food. The bird tries to swallow seeds but, because of the thick deposits on the mucous membrane of the gullet, does not succeed.

Incidence and prognosis: Crop congestion is not a common disease. It can persist over a period of weeks before the bird dies of emaciation and blood poisoning. Treatment of the disease is only successful if commenced within a few days of the appearance of the symptoms described above.

Therapy: The bird is given one drop of 0.1-0.2% aqueous solution of hydrochloric acid into the beak (with a pipette) three times a day. Hydrochloric acid prevents the formation of abnormal fermentation acids. Instead of its drinking water, the patient receives warm chamomile tea to which Aureomycin has been added. An infra-red radiator is placed inside the cage and left on day and night.

Intestinal Inflammation (Enteritis)

Cause: It is convenient to differentiate between infectious inflammation of the intestinal mucosa caused by living agents (bacteria, coccidians, worms) and non-infectious types caused by the widest possible range of adverse factors. The latter occur most commonly and are largely traced back to chills and deficient nutrition.

The most important infectious diseases of the intestine in small birds are paratyphoid infections and coccidiosis. They are discussed under the appropriate headings.

Clinical picture and diagnosis: A bird suffering from a mild intestinal inflammation is quieter than usual and fluffs up its feathers slightly when feeling unobserved. If the condition grows worse, the bird looks like a ball of feathers, listlessly sifts through its seed cup, and – because of the severe loss of fluid – drinks a great deal. The rear end of the body is often bloated, hot, and reddened, and during the frequent voiding of droppings the bird sometimes moves the tail up and down. The vent feathers are wet and matted with liquid feces. The consistency of the droppings may be tough and sticky, gruel-like or broth-like, or watery. The color may be grayish brown or – if blood is present – dark brown or blackish red. A foul odor is not uncommon. The duration of enteritis varies greatly.

Incidence and prognosis: Particularly at risk from enteritis are freshly caught and newly imported birds, and a large proportion of these birds still die of this disease today. A large consignment of birds that has just arrived after a long journey almost always includes a few animals affected with intestinal inflammation. If treatment is commenced early, most cases of avian enteritis can now be cured, thanks to the modern drugs at our disposal.

Treatment: A bird suffering from enteritis should be isolated immediately if not already kept in a cage of its own. It should drink water that has been boiled and to which an antibiotic has been added. Oxytetracycline (Terramycin) and chlortetracycline (Aureomycin) have proved successful, either on their own or combined with vitamins. Codrinal is effective against intestinal inflammation caused by coccidian infections, as is Supronal, a sulfonamide administered at four drops to 30 ccm water. In weaver finches suffering from intestinal disease, a quick cure has repeatedly been achieved with vitamins of the B complex. Large doses of vitamin B preparations and the antibiotics mentioned above have no adverse effects on these birds.

Apart from drug treatment, the bird is also hastened on the

THE WORLD'S LARGEST SELECTION OF PET, ANIMAL, AND MUSIC BOOKS.

T.F.H. Publications publishes more than 900 books covering many hobby aspects (dogs, cats, birds, fish, small animals, music, etc.). Whether you are a beginner or an advanced hobbyist you will find exactly what you're looking for among our complete listing of books. For a free catalog fill out the form on the other side of this page and mail it today.

.. CATS ...

... BIRDS ..

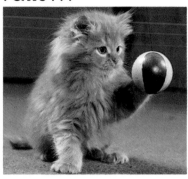

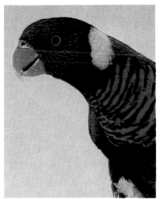

... ANIMALS ...

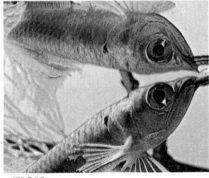

... DOGS ...

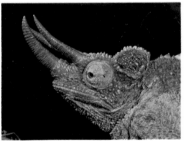

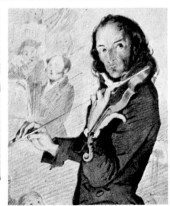

.. FISH ...

... MUSIC ...

For more than 30 years, *Tropical Fish Hobbyist* has been the source of accurate, up-to-the-minute, and fascinating information on every facet of the aquarium hobby.

Join the more than 50,000 devoted readers worldwide who wouldn't miss a single issue.

road to recovery by an unvaryingly warm environment of about 35°C, which is most easily maintained by means of an infra-red radiator that is switched on day and night. If this type of radiator is not available, one can make do with a hot-water bottle carefully wrapped and laid on the bottom of the cage, while keeping the cage covered with a cloth. In the winter the cage is placed (with caution!) near the heater. Diseases of the intestine may also be treated in a special hospital cage heated with light bulbs under a metal grate.

Constipation

Cause: Constipation can develop after the ingestion of food which is difficult to digest. As a result of this food, hardened fecal matter accumulates inside the ceca and the cloaca.

Clinical picture and diagnosis: The bird sits about with fluffed-up feathers, eats little or nothing, and occasionally makes pushing movements with the tail.

Incidence: Constipation is a very rare condition in our cage birds. In females it must not be confused with egg binding.

Therapy: With the aid of a pipette, the bird is given a few drops of castor oil, mineral oil, or olive oil into the beak. Alternatively, warmed oil may be sprayed into the cloaca with the pipette. As drinking water the patient receives Glauber's salt (sodium sulphate) in a solution of 1:200.

Swallowed Foreign Bodies

The assumption that the wild bird instinctively swallows only what is good for it is a fallacy. Insect- and worm-eating species frequently swallow foreign bodies such as rubber bands, pieces of wire, shoe laces, and bits of string which they perhaps mistake for something edible because of the worm-like shape. Such indigestible objects are often excreted with the feces, but sometimes—because of their nature or shape—the intestinal musculature cannot move them on. Then they cause the bird's death. They obstruct the intestinal lumen, produce an invagination of the intestine (intussusception), or injure the intestinal mucosa through stricture. Pieces of wire and pins that have been swallowed pierce the gastric or intestinal wall and cause a purulent peritonitis.

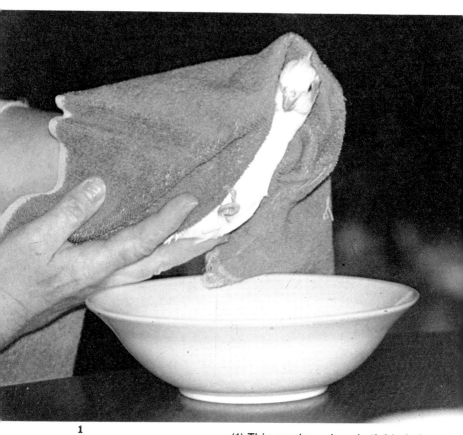

1

(1) This egg-bound cockatiel is being held over steaming water to aid expulsion of the egg. (2) This cage is well suited to a cockatoo. It is large enough to allow the bird to stretch its wings and strong enough to prevent it from breaking out. When the cage is positioned in a window, it is important that the bird does not receive the direct rays of the sun or a draft.

2 →

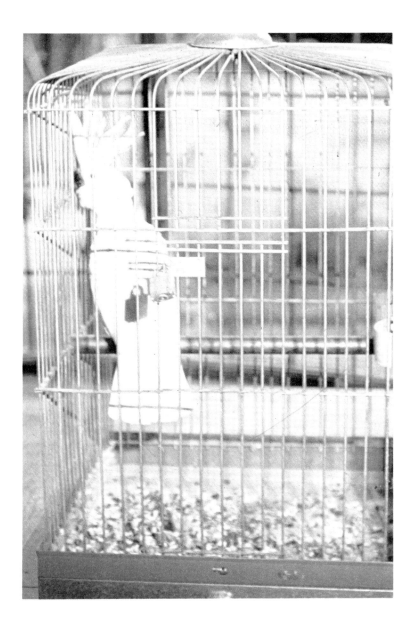

Whether this type of behavior springs from playful motives or mistakes is not known. Particularly at risk are birds which are allowed to fly about inside the house. Before opening the cage door, one should always make sure that no string, rubber bands, or pins are lying about.

A bird that has swallowed a foreign body suffers from vague ill health, takes in little food, and grows progressively weaker until days or weeks later death ensues. There are cases, however, which end in a cure through expulsion of the foreign body. Thus a shama which had been ill for three weeks suddenly brought up a full-size shoe lace compressed into a ball, and from that moment it was in perfect health again. It has also happened that the keeper suddenly saw one end of a piece of string sticking out of the bird's anus while the bird was pushing with all its might, and succeeded in removing the foreign body by pulling it out very slowly and carefully.

Where a bird has been seen to swallow a foreign body, one can try to encourage the passage through the intestinal canal by dropping mineral oil or olive oil into the bird's beak.

RESPIRATORY SYSTEM
Structure of the Respiratory Organs

The respiratory organs of birds are fundamentally different from those of mammals. They have become entirely adapted to the great workload necessitated by flying.

In addition to the larynx—which it has in common with mammals—the bird has a syrinx, the voice-box proper. While the larynx in birds is used for respiration, the syrinx—situated at the lower end of the trachea—is the vocal organ which produces sound and song.

Avian lungs consist of two rigid lobes which are firmly attached at the sides. The lung tissue is composed of a complex system of tubes. The two main bronchi extending from the syrinx split into a greatly ramified bronchial system and eventually into a network of air capillaries. These air capillaries closely interweave with a very fine network of blood capillaries from the pulmonary arteries to form the true respiratory tissue in which the gaseous exchange between air and blood takes place.

One of the most important prerequisites for flight is lightness.

The birds have solved this problem, among other ways, by an extensive distribution of bronchi or air sacs. These thin walled and elastic structures are found everywhere in the body, even extending into the bones of the wings, the breastbone, and the subcutaneous tissue. Because of the way the air sacs are constructed, the inspired air can be utilized much more efficiently than is possible with the mammalian respiratory system. These air sacs are directly linked to the greater and lesser bronchi and serve not only as an air reservoir but also as an organ of ventilation. Since the bird, with its intense metabolism and high body temperature, does not possess sweat glands, the air sacs carry out this heat-regulatory function.

Congestion of the Respiratory Passages

Cause: Congestion of the respiratory passages in the bird corresponds to the common cold in man and is precipitated by the same factors — that is, chills through drafts or sudden changes in temperature.

Clinical picture: The affected bird sneezes frequently and in rapid succession, sounding to the human ear roughly like "pfft-pfft-pfft," accompanied by nodding the head. At the same time a watery or slimy fluid is disposed of by violent head-shaking. Because the nasal cavities are blocked, the bird breathes with the beak open. Where the illness continues over a longer period the upper surface of the tongue dries up (because of the permanently open beak) and develops a membranous deposit of a whitish color. In the past this abnormality of the tongue, known as "pips" among breeders, was remedied by the barbarous method of scraping it off with a sharp knife. This method is ineffective and, if anything, worsens the course of the disease. In fowl, colds lead to swellings above and below the eyes which are often so severe that the eyes look like mere slits. The swellings are due to the upper and lower chambers of the eye filling up with secretion. In song birds, congestion presents the further symptoms of hoarseness and temporarily complete loss of voice.

Incidence and prognosis: Congestion of the respiratory passages is fairly common in our cage and aviary birds. It is usually caused by drafts resulting from the simultaneous opening of windows and doors, as when the housewife is doing her spring cleaning

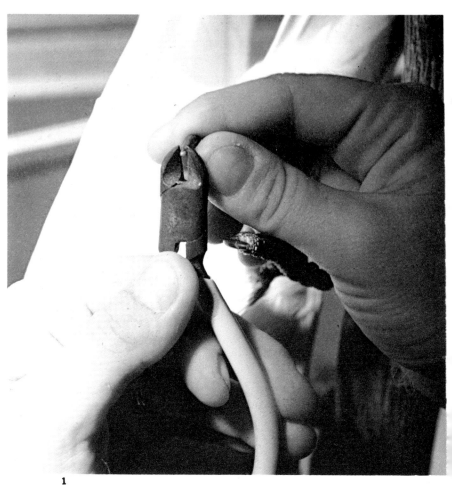

1

Trimming a bird's claws must be done carefully
so that the blood vessel that runs partway into
each claw is not severed. (1) Trimming the claws
of a large parrot is usually a two-man operation,
with one person holding the bird while the other
does the trimming. (2) One person is able to trim
a small bird's claws. If you are unsure of the
proper procedure for claw trimming, have your
veterinarian or some other experienced person
show you how it is done.

2 →

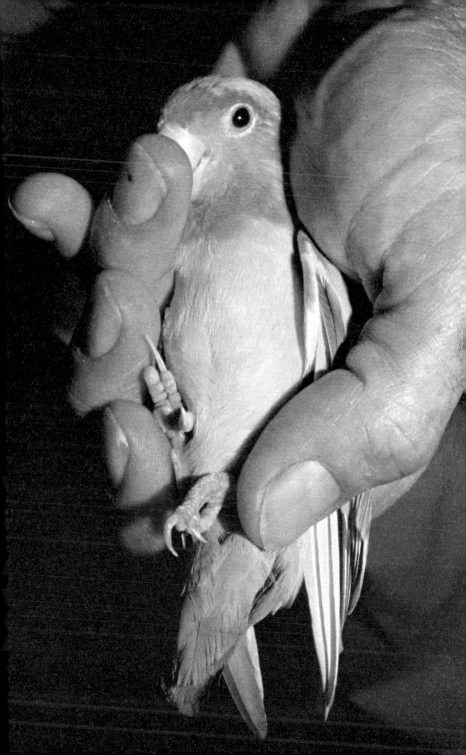

and the cage stands in the middle of the aired room unprotected by a cover. Among the inhabitants of outdoor aviaries, delicate finches such as Gouldian finches and other waxbills catch colds very easily when sudden drops in temperature occur which are combined with rain showers. During the molting period all birds are very susceptible to colds. The chances of a recovery are good, provided treatment is started early.

Treatment: Birds suffering from colds are subjected to radiation with an infra-red radiator until all symptoms of the cold have cleared up. In addition, the patient receives tepid drinking water to which an antibiotic (Aureomycin, Terramycin) has been added.

Pneumonia

Cause: The causes of pneumonia are the same as those of congestion of the respiratory passages. If the bird is exposed to these adverse environmental factors for long enough, pneumonia develops. Apart from being incited by drafts and temperature changes, pneumonia may also result from the clumsy administration of liquid medicines which enter the trachea and from infectious diseases such as mycosis and paratyphoid.

Clinical picture: Birds suffering from pneumonia sit on the perch or the bottom of the cage with fluffed-up feathers. Their breathing is labored, with the beak opening and shutting rhythmically and whistling and rustling noises being heard. Sometimes the patient rids itself of yellowish mucus, flinging it away by shaking its head about.

Incidence and prognosis: Pneumonia is frequently observed in freshly imported birds, which often suffer from some form of intestinal inflammation at the same time. The chances of a recovery are slim because affected birds usually develop severe congestion of the lungs (pulmonary edema) as a result of circulatory weakness.

Treatment: The patient receives heat treatment from an infrared radiator, plus an antibiotic into the beak (given with a pipette). Better still, the antibiotic is injected into the pectoral musculature. To support the circulation, a heart-strengthening drug may be employed.

REPRODUCTIVE ORGANS
Egg-binding

Cause: Egg-binding, the bird's inability to expel the egg from the oviduct, has a variety of causes. Many cases of egg-binding are due to the egg lacking a firm calcium shell. Only the hard-shelled egg has the ability to go with the pressures of oviductal and abdominal musculature and move toward the cloaca. An egg protected by only a delicate membrane does nothing to escape from the pressure exerted by the muscle contractions that are designed to propel it. If responding at all, it elastically alters its shape and merely glides to and fro without allowing itself to be expelled.

Clinical picture and diagnosis: The hen suffering from egg-binding crouches on the floor with the feathers fluffed out and the eyes closed, looking seriously ill. The area around the vent is swollen, with the skin reddened and hot. From time to time straining movements are made, as if the hen were trying to void droppings. Whenever these symptoms are observed in a breeding hen, egg-binding is certain to be the cause.

Incidence and prognosis: In bird breeding, egg-binding is one of the most common diseases of the hen. Soft-shelled eggs are produced mainly by species with intense laying activity such as gamebirds (quail, pheasants), certain weaver finches (striated finch, white-rumped mannikin, zebra finch, and cut-throat finch), and many species of doves (collared turtle dove, diamond dove, bleeding heart dove). Unless the breeder removes the cock in good time, the females continue to lay eggs until they are utterly exhausted. In such cases the female cannot meet the persistently high calcium requirements quickly enough and we get egg-binding due to soft-shelled eggs as a result. In weaver finches, a sudden change in the temperature very often brings on egg-binding. If the birds are transferred from a warm room to outdoor aviaries in the spring, or from outdoor aviaries to a warm room in the fall, many hens promptly come to suffer from egg-binding. In all species, young hens often have laying difficulties with regard to their first egg because the oviduct is not yet sufficiently elastic.

Treatment: When a hen is suffering from egg-binding, one

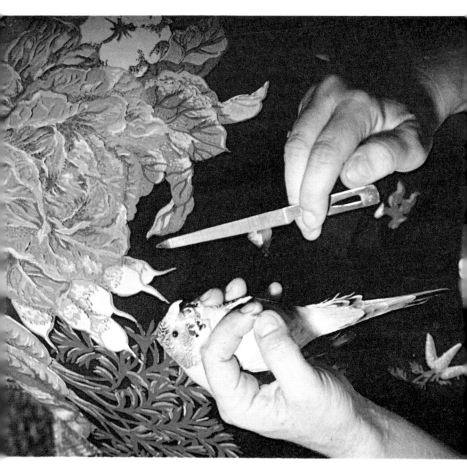

1

(1) Instead of, or in addition to, nail clippers, a file can be used to shape overgrown beaks and claws. (2) By nibbling at the cuttlebone, these cockatiels wear their beaks down naturally.

2 →

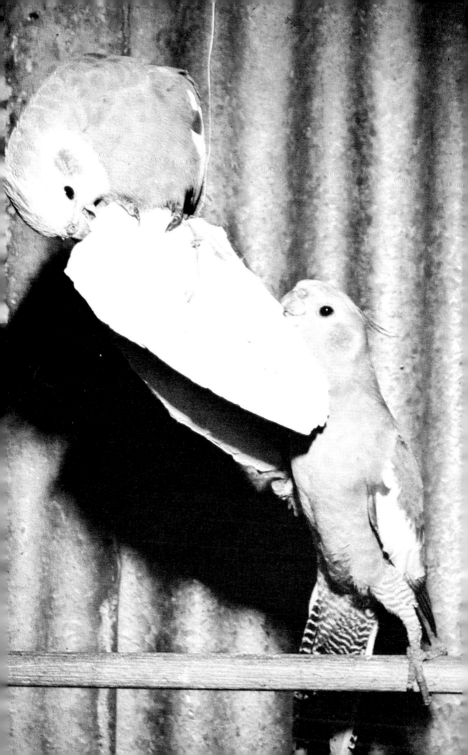

checks carefully whether the obstruction is caused by a soft-shelled egg or a normal one. Soft-shelled eggs are squashed by careful pressure with the fingers, and the pieces usually appear without much delay. If the egg is felt to have a hard shell, however, one refrains from squashing it since the hard edges of the shell could injure the mucous membrane of the oviduct. With the aid of a thin pipette, one inserts a drop of cod-liver oil, olive oil, or mineral oil into the cloaca and then treats the patient with infra-red radiation. Where this method is employed, the egg usually appears within half an hour, and that is precisely how long the bird needs to recover. A hospital cage heated from the bottom with light bulbs achieves the same result. If neither of these heat sources is available, the hen's cage is covered with a cloth which has previously been immersed in hot water and then wrung out. Take care, however, that the bird is not suffocated by excessively hot steam.

Egg-binding can largely be prevented by a diet which is rich in calcium. If the seeds are slightly moistened with fresh cod-liver oil so that only a thin film of oil envelops them, the birds are happy to accept this food. This method has been used successfully by breeders of weaver finches. As breeding hens of these species are highly sensitive to fluctuations in temperature, the breeder should ensure that the temperature remains as constant as possible, and in the fall he should avoid transferring his birds to very warm rooms. In spring the birds should only be moved into outdoor aviaries in warm weather. If the indoor compartment of the aviary is equipped with an infra-red radiator, the birds can keep themselves sufficiently warm even when sudden drops in temperature occur.

NERVOUS SYSTEM
Cerebral Concussion

Concussion of the brain resulting from accidents is one of the most common causes of death in cage and aviary birds. Cerebral concussion is sustained when the flying bird collides with hard surfaces such as glass panes, taut wire mesh, and iron frames in the aviary. Many budgerigars which are allowed regular free flights in the home have fatal accidents because they do not recognize well-cleaned windows as obstacles. The budgie is in fact particularly prone to accidents of this type. If birds of this species are startled out of their sleep in the night by unknown sounds, light from flashlights, or by cats running about on the aviary roof, they rush off into the dark in a panic and bump into the aviary wire. These birds, whose natural environment is most often plains or prairies, are simply not "programmed" to allow for obstacles when it comes to their flight behavior.

A bird which has bumped head-on into an obstacle drops to the ground and at first lies there as though unconscious. Depending on the severity of the impact and the extent of brain damage involved, the animal may recover once the shock has worn off or it may remain on the ground with paralysis of the legs and disturbances of balance. Externally the bird seldom looks injured in any way, which means the keeper is confronted by a mystery if he has not seen the accident happen.

On dissection, a bird that has died of cerebral concussion usually shows areas of bleeding in the meninges (lining of the brain) and rarely injuries to the bones of the skull or hemorrhages inside the brain tissue.

There is no known treatment for concussion of the brain in the bird. The method usually recommended in the literature is to move the bird to a dark and cool place, certainly a kind-hearted act but unlikely to bring any real relief to the sick animal. There is only one thing we can do with such a bird, and that is to wait and see. One bird may recover when the shock has worn off, while another dies hours or days after the accident.

The signs of a cerebral concussion frequently resemble those of vitamin B deficiency. The two conditions can, however, be differentiated because a bird suffering from vitamin deficiency will usually have had attacks of weakness and disturbances of balance before the first seizure, whereas a bird with cerebral concussion will have been completely healthy.

To prevent accidents, the glass walls of cages and aviaries should be made visible by being marked with a little whitewash. The wire mesh of the outdoor flight must not be too taut, but should be slack enough to "give" when a bird flies into it. The wire mesh should also be fastened below the iron framework so the birds do not fly into these hard surfaces and sustain head injuries.

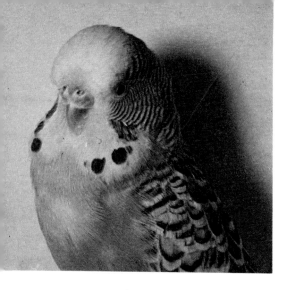

Tumors are sometimes caused by defects in nutrition. **Left:** There is a high incidence of tumors in budgerigars. **Below:** Pigeons and doves rarely develop tumors.

Vitamin Deficiencies and Poisons

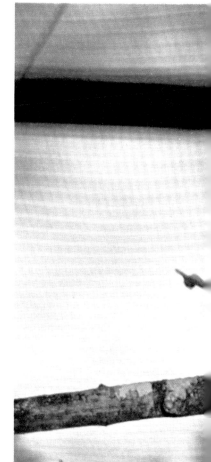

Vitamins are organic compounds of a complex structure which are present in foods either fully formed or in a precursory state. They are required by the body in very small quantities but are absolutely vital for the maintenance of health and the individual's ability to function normally. Vitamins regulate the utilization of substances required by the body for growth and nutrition, such as fats, proteins, carbohydrates, and minerals. Each vitamin has a specific function which cannot be fulfilled in the same way by any other vitamin. If a vitamin is absent from the diet, the body responds with signs of disease—though often not until weeks have elapsed—which will end in death if the missing substance is

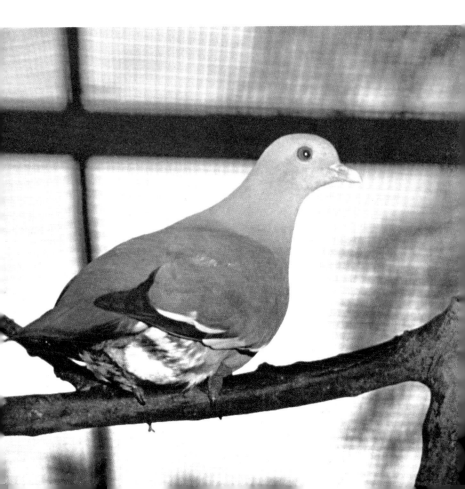

not supplied. Since many diseases produced by a deficiency or absence of a particular vitamin run a fairly characteristic course, it is often not too difficult to identify the vitamin concerned. Where treatment is started in the early stages, the bird's life can usually be saved.

The absence of some vitamins from our foodstuffs is explained by the sensitivity of these substances and the fact that they are rapidly destroyed by high temperatures and atmospheric oxygen. Above all, vitamin B_1, pantothenic acid, the carotenes, and vitamins A, D, and E quickly lose their effectiveness if a foodstuff is stored for any length of time. In the numerous vitamin preparations available on the market, the sensitive substances are stabilized in a variety of ways, which makes them keep for long periods. Nonetheless, all vitamin preparations should be stored in a dark and cool place.

Where a bird shows certain characteristic signs of vitamin deficiency, it is advisable to treat it by administering the vitamin concerned in high doses until a cure has been effected. Most vitamins are tolerated well by the organism at very high dosages, even at a thousand times the amount considered to be the daily requirement. Exceptions are vitamins A and D. Here the administration of large quantities over long periods can result in the appearance of symptoms signifying a disease known as hypervitaminosis.

Vitamin deficiency diseases are of much more common occurrence in cage birds than is generally supposed by the keeper. In most cases, however, the symptoms are not interpreted correctly and the bird is sentenced to death. Below I shall describe those aspects of the functions of vitamins as are of relevance to the bird fancier and describe the disease symptoms occurring in the bird when certain vitamins are lacking.

VITAMIN A DEFICIENCY

Function: Vitamin A is required for the normal growth of the feathers and for the health and proper functioning of the mucous membranes.

Clinical picture: In cases of vitamin A deficiency a clear clinical picture is not always present. Characteristic are the abnormalities seen with regard to the eye. At first there is a swelling of the conjunctiva combined with tears in the eyes; later the cornea grows opaque; and eventually the eye keratinizes and disintegrates. Bald headedness of certain passerine birds and inflammations of the feet in insectivores resulting from feeding excessive quantities of mealworms are likely to stem from vitamin A deficiency as well.

Incidence and prognosis: Blindness in cage birds due to a diet deficient in vitamin A is observed most frequently in weaver finches, particularly *Erythrura* species. Baldness of the head and neck, so common in many species of weaver finches, is rapidly cured by moving the birds to outdoor aviaries. In this case the carotene (vitamin A precursor) ingested in large amounts with green plant food is obviously responsible for the quick growth of new feathers. In some cases where the beak had grown crosswise or abnormally long, an addition of vitamin A to the diet achieved a normal growth of the horny beak. Since this vitamin checks the excessive growth of the horny substance, vitamin A therapy is always indicated in cases of exaggerated growth of the beak and claws. The prognosis is good as long as the eye changes have not yet led to keratinization of the cornea or the skin of the head does not already look completely keratinized and mummified.

Treatment: The bird is given one drop of pure vitamin A per day into the angle of the beak with a pipette. Treatment is continued until a cure has been achieved. Your veterinarian will advise you as to the best vitamin supplement. As a preventive measure, the birds are given fresh green plant food whenever possible. Chlorophyll, the substance responsible for the green color of the leaves, contains plenty of betacarotene, the most important precursor of vitamin A. Many weaver finches at first refuse green plant food, but they soon learn to accept it when small containers with chickweed or spiderwort are put inside the cage. Insectivores get their supply of carotene if we moisten their soft food with grated carrot.

VITAMIN B DEFICIENCY

Disease signs: Epilepsy, vertigo, fits, giddiness, and mental symptoms are characteristic.

Cause: The vitamins of the B complex consist of a range of organic compounds which vary considerably from each other in

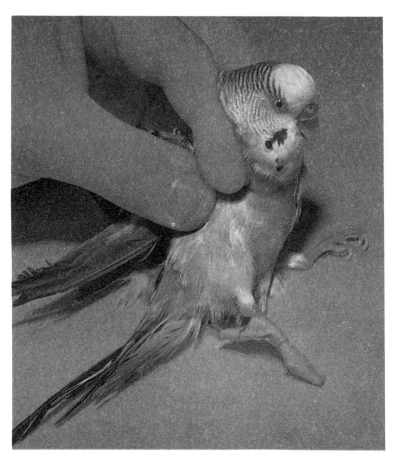

1

(1) Since fractures heal so quickly in birds, this budgerigar's splint can be removed in about two weeks. (2) There is no cure known for the lumps caused by ingrowing feathers on this Norwich canary. (3) This budgerigar has a disorder of the nervous system known as St. Vitus's dance, or chorea. Irregular, jerking movements are caused by involuntary muscle contractions.

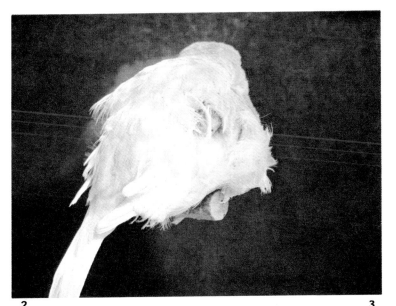

2

3

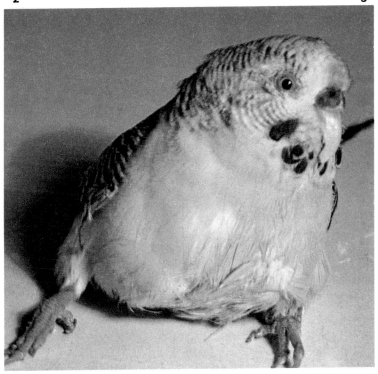

their composition, the only common factor being that they have all been isolated from yeast. Belonging to the B group are vitamin B_1 (aneurin, thiamin), vitamin B_2 (riboflavin), pantothenic acid, nicotinamide, biotin, vitamin B_6 (pyridoxine), folic acid, and vitamin B_{12} (cobalamin). The functions of most B vitamins in the metabolism are known: they are important constituents of enzyme systems in the body which control all the chemical changes.

Vitamin B deficiency is without a doubt the most common cause of deficiency diseases in cage birds. As regards its signs and symptoms, it is also the most striking one.

Clinical picture: It never fails to astonish one how little even experienced bird fanciers know about the origin of fits and seizures occurring in their pets. The early signs of the disease are generally overlooked or misinterpreted. Initially the bird grows conspicuously lethargic and suffers from a weakness of the legs, because of which it likes to rest on the perch with the abdomen, thus taking the weight off the legs. Jumps from perch to perch are undertaken reluctantly and clumsily. When sitting, the bird tends to fall over—either backward or head first—and struggles to maintain its equilibrium by flapping with the wings. Take-off is reasonably successful, but when the bird has landed, it staggers to the seed and water cups as though drunk. The disturbances of balance grow progressively worse, the head is rotated, and one day the first fit takes place. The bird tries to hold on to the perch with its claws while hanging head downward and beating with the wings. Eventually it lets go and crash-lands on the bottom of the cage, where it somersaults a few times and at last—keeping its balance by holding the wings spread out and resting them on the cage bottom—sits still, exhausted. After a rest the bird may be able to hop back onto the perch as though perfectly healthy. These attacks repeat themselves at increasingly shorter intervals and may continue over a period of many months until death. They can easily be provoked in the bird through excitement, even by feeding the bird and cleaning the cage.

Paralysis of the legs is not uncommonly seen in budgerigars between seven and nine weeks of age. This disease, with spasms of the toes in the absence of a deformity, is caused by vitamin B_1 (riboflavin) deficiency.

That intestinal inflammations can also be connected with vitamin B deficiency is shown by the successful treatment of newly imported Gouldian finches from Japan. These birds were suffering from enteritis but were cured by the administration of vitamin B_{12} (cobalamin).

Incidence and prognosis: The fits and seizures caused by a deficiency of vitamins of the B group can affect all groups of birds. Experience has shown, however, that they are most common in starlings, finches, shrikes, and birds of prey. The high incidence of this deficiency disease in caged birds is largely due to the fact that these vitamins are readily destroyed in the food.

Treatment should start as early as possible and will then, as a rule, be successful. Disturbances of the equilibrium and early fits quickly clear up when high doses of vitamins of the B complex are given. Where the patient has been suffering from attacks for months, it is too late for a complete cure although an improvement may still be achieved. At this late stage the extremely sensitive nervous tissue can no longer regenerate itself sufficiently.

Somewhat similar to the symptoms of vitamin B deficiency are those of cerebral concussion. Fits and paralysis of the legs caused by concussion have a very sudden onset, however.

Vitamin E deficiency, which is much rarer, also produces some of the signs seen in vitamin B deficiency: weakness of the legs, lack of coordination when hopping from perch to perch, and an abnormal posture of the head (holding the head well to the side or downward). Where one is not certain about the nature of the disease, treatment with vitamins of the B complex should be carried out in any case. To patients suffering from weakness of the legs, vitamin E should be administered in addition.

Treatment: A preparation should be used which contains all the vitamins of the B complex. While the fits appear to be precipitated mainly by a deficiency of vitamins B_1, B_2, and B_6, there may be other components which are also absent. Numerous B-complex preparations are available on the market and from your veterinarian. These drugs can be administered in drop form or as tablets (put in water and stirred into a pulp). In severe cases they can also be injected into the pectoral musculature. Treatment by administering the drug with a pipette is required several times a day, in some cases perhaps

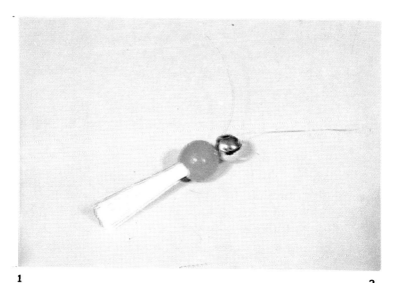

1

2

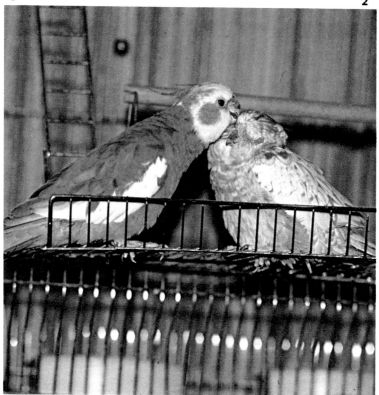

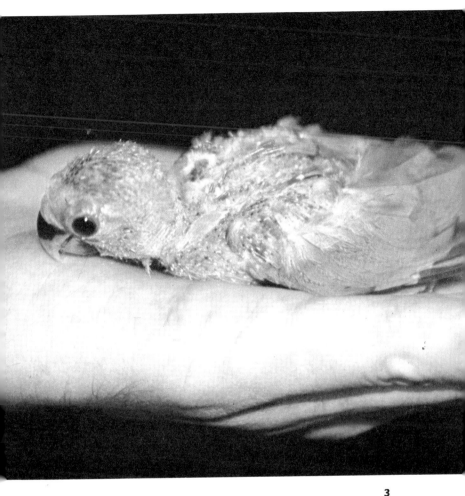

3

(1) Hanging toys in a bird's cage will often help to amuse your bird, and they may serve to prevent or alleviate feather plucking. (2) Preening and mating activities are sometimes the cause of feather loss in one or the other of the pair. New feathers usually grow in quickly. (3) This lovebird chick has been severely feather-plucked. Once the chick is able to feed itself and is separated from its parents, it should feather out normally.

even at three-hour intervals. The patient will come to no harm if the dosage is exceeded.

Fits and seizures due to vitamin B deficiency can also occur in sick birds which have been treated with sulfonamides for too long, since these chemicals seriously deplete the body's vitamin store. For this reason every course of treatment with sulfonamides should be followed by a course of treatment with multivitamins.

One excellent source of B vitamins is dried yeast, the only vitamin of the B group it does not contain being cobalamin (vitamin B_{12}). Regular additions of yeast to the food prevent vitamin B deficiency.

VITAMIN D DEFICIENCY

Function: Vitamin D is required for the normal growth of the skeleton. The vitamin makes possible the ossification and growth of the bones, and it promotes the resorption of calcium from the intestine and prevents its excretion in the feces. More generally, vitamin D regulates the phosphorus and calcium metabolism of the body. Vitamin D deficiency occurs as rickets in young animals and as osteomalacia in adult birds, both forms of osteoporosis.

Clinical picture: Young birds affected with rickets show severe curvature of the calcium-deficient bones. As a result, they at first suffer from lameness, then grow knock-kneed, and in the later stages are merely able to crouch on their joints. In adult birds, osteoporosis (osteomalacia) is seen most frequently in hens with a high laying activity and a diet which is low in calcium. The body mobilizes calcium stored in the bones in order to use it for egg-shell production. In numerous cases this eventually results in the laying of eggs without shells. Since these cannot, as a rule, leave the oviduct, egg-binding sets in.

Incidence and prognosis: In the past, rickets was fairly common among young birds reared in captivity. Nowadays the condition has become rare since even the inexperienced keeper is generally aware of the birds' need for calcium in the food. Where the toes are already crippled and the feet are in an abnormal ("bandy-legged") position, a course of vitamin D comes too late to correct the extremities. While the bones ossify, they still maintain their abnormal position. The still fairly pliable legs and toes of young birds may resume their normal position with the aid of splints.

Treatment: Of the various D vitamins, vitamin D_3 has the greatest effect on skeletal growth in the bird. It is contained in fish oil but is most easily obtainable in supplements, especially the preparation known as Vigantol. Unlike most vitamins, D must be fed cautiously as an overdose has serious side effects.

VITAMIN E DEFICIENCY

Cause: Vitamin E is a decisive factor in intermediary metabolic processes of the body. Further, it acts as an antioxidant. It reduces the oxygen requirements in the tissues and thereby protects other sensitive vitamins, as well as hormones and enzymes, from destruction by the action of oxygen. In addition, it promotes the function and growth of the musculature and—via the pituitary gland (hypophysis)—regulates the function of the reproductive organs. In the bird, vitamin E deficiency expresses itself most noticeably through disturbances in the nervous system (encephalomalacia) and a poor hatching rate of young birds from the eggs.

Clinical picture: The bird is lethargic and drowsy in the early stages, as well as clumsy in its movements, and only hops from perch to perch very reluctantly. Later mild disturbances of the equilibrium add to the signs, gradually growing more marked as the weeks and months go by. The bird now shows uncoordinated movements and constantly turns the head sideways or moves it down to the abdomen. In the terminal stage of the disease, complete paralysis sets in.

The absence of vitamin E from the food is explained by the fact that this substance is very sensitive to oxidation and hence of very limited life in storage.

Incidence and prognosis: The above symptoms have been observed on a regular basis in birds of paradise in a zoo. That identical or similar E-deficiency phenomena can occur in other bird species as well is virtually certain. (Deficiency symptoms were in fact first identified in domestic chickens.) Vitamin E supplements administered at regular intervals brought to an abrupt halt the mortality among birds of paradise in the Dutch zoological garden and effected a complete cure.

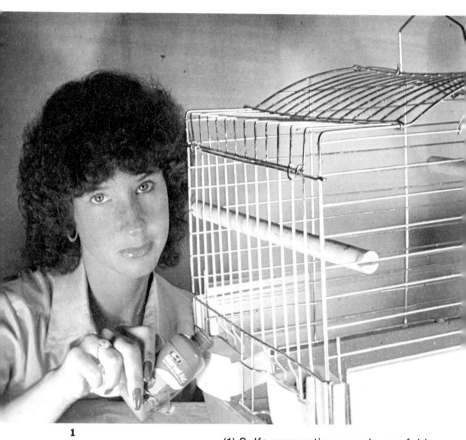

1

(1) Sulfa preparations can be useful in countering gastrointestinal illness. (2) This cockatiel is being fed vitamins with an eyedropper.

2 →

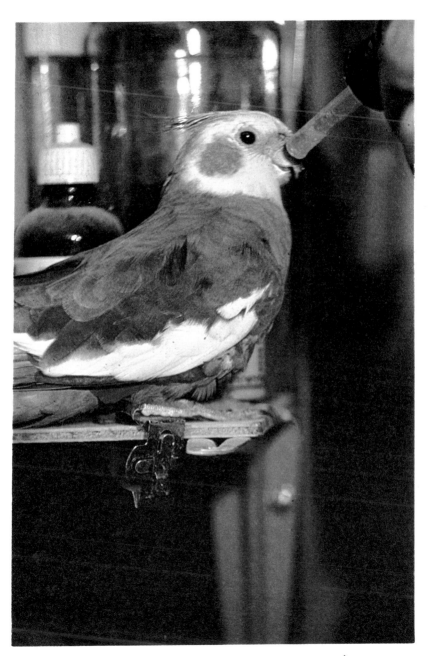

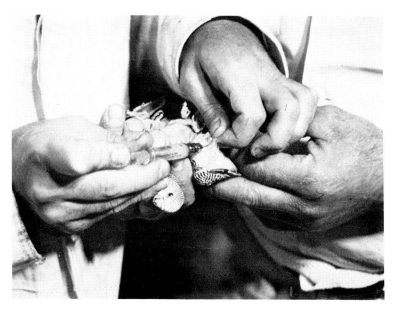
Administration of medication by injection should be attempted only by professionals or thoroughly experienced persons.

Therapy: Vitamin E is present in large amounts in wheat-germ oil from which the chemically active compound tocopherol has been isolated. It is available on the market as several stabilized vitamin E preparations.

POISONS
Insecticide Poisoning
The application of contact insecticides for the destruction of parasites in cages and aviaries frequently leads to cases of poisoning among the birds. Since the toxic effect such an insecticide has on warm-blooded animals is dependent on the amount and concentration in which it is used, it is absolutely vital that the stated dosage be strictly adhered to. On no account must insecticides in oily solution be employed, as the toxic substance deeply penetrates the tissues together with the oil, causing severe poisoning. Less dangerous are insecticides in an aqueous solution or in powder form. Unfortunate experiences in aviaries and bird rooms have also been had with insecticides applied in the form of sprays and vapors. As a result of inhaling the toxic

fumes, hummingbirds and other small birds fell in mid-flight. Larger birds which have swallowed insects sprayed with insecticide come to suffer from incurable paralysis of the legs, making it necessary for them to be put to sleep.

Before taking any action involving insecticides, remove all the birds from the cages and aviaries. Air the housing very thoroughly before reintroducing the birds. Food and water cups should be cleaned thoroughly before their reuse.

Not infrequently, keepers have also reported cases of poisoning caused by lettuce that had been sprayed. Such lettuce cannot be rendered safe even if washed thoroughly or steeped in water for hours before use. The cautious keeper would do better to give chickweed or spiderwort grown in his own garden to his birds instead.

Ergotism

Ergot is the resistant form of a parasitic fungus *(Claviceps purpurea)* growing on the young seed heads of grasses. It forms cylindrical three-edged granules which are blackish violet in color. Among the grasses grown for bird seeds, canary seed *(Phalaris canariensis)* is frequently affected. On this plant the mycotic granules grow no bigger than the canary seeds themselves.

Ergotism has been known to occur in Gouldian finches and other finches *(Spermestes)* which eat a lot of canary seed. Affected birds suffer from forms of paralysis which end fatally. The ingestion of a minute ergot particle is sufficient for poisoning to occur. Particularly dangerous is mycotic canary seed which has been soaked in water as a raising-food for young weaver finches. In fowl the ingestion of very small quantities of ergot causes necrosis of the toe joints, a fairly characteristic symptom which has not yet been observed in song birds.

When seed-eaters exhibit sudden paralysis, the keeper should carefully examine the seeds for the presence of ergot. This fungus is one reason why the purchase of cheap seeds which have not been cleaned must be avoided! Just like the cereals intended for human consumption, canary seeds can be freed from ergot by being machine-cleaned.

The antidote recommended in cases of ergotism is tannin.

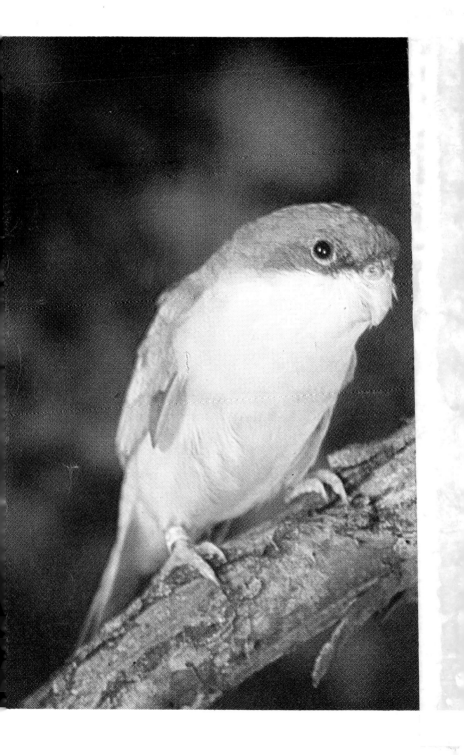